Andreas Vesalius

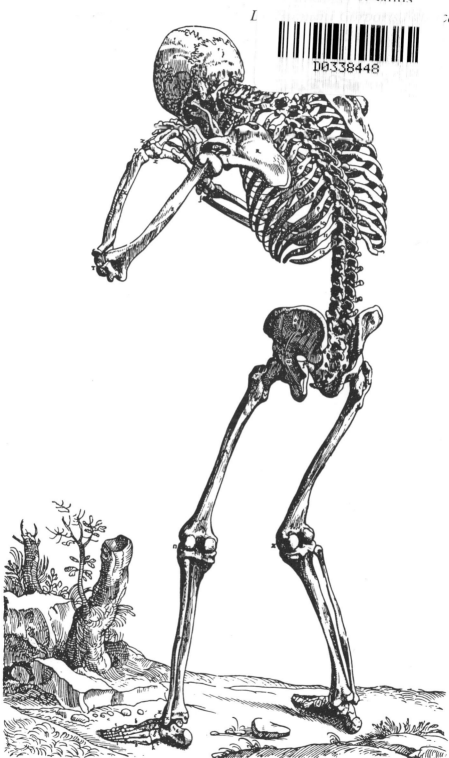

The Chiropractic Theories

A Synopsis of Scientific Research

Second Edition

The Chiropractic Theories

A Synopsis of Scientific Research

Second Edition

Robert A. Leach, AA, DC, FICC

Chairman, Mississippi Associated Chiropractors Committee on Research
Private general practice of chiropractic

with contribution from

Reed B. Phillips, DC, MSCM, DACBR, FICC

Postgraduate Extension Faculty,
  Los Angeles Chiropractic College
  Western States Chiropractic College
President, American Chiropractic Board of Roentgenology Examining Board
Chairman, Research Committee of the American Chiropractic College of
  Roentgenology
Secretary, Radiology Section of the American Public Health Association
Private practice of chiropractic roentgenology

illustrated by Robert S. Fritzius, BS

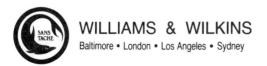

WILLIAMS & WILKINS
Baltimore • London • Los Angeles • Sydney

Editor: Jonathan W. Pine, Jr.
Associate Editor: Victoria M. Vaughn
Copy editor: Bill Cady
Design: Bert Smith
Illustration Planning: Reginald R. Stanley
Production: Raymond E. Reter

Printed in the United States of America

First Edition, 1980

Library of Congress Cataloging in Publication Data

Leach, Robert A.
    The chiropractic theories.

    Bibliography: p.
    Includes index.
    1. Chiropractic—Philosophy. 2. Joints—Dislocations. I. Phillips, Reed B. II.
Title: RZ242.L42 1986   615.5'34   85-9491
    ISBN 0-683-04906-2

Composed and printed at the
Waverly Press, Inc.

85 86 87 88 89
10 9 8 7 6 5 4 3 2 1

To Vicki, whose ubiquitous nature permits the raising of our family and the continuation of this work, I am forever indebted.

Foreword

Inasmuch as chiropractic lays claim to be one of the health professions, it also lays claim to a body of knowledge, not simply a body of therapeutic techniques. Where such knowledge is systemized, consistent, coherent, communicable and researchable, it is legitimate to speak of chiropractic as a health discipline.

This requires, however, much more than the mere incorporation of the basic sciences, and elements of other health sciences, into the chiropractic paradigm. A profession must be committed not only to the application of knowledge in the service of humankind but also to the creation and dissemination of new knowledge. This requires a cadre of active scholars who are committed, through whatever means, such as philosophical reflection or empirical research, to grappling with the major intellectual puzzles of the discipline.

It is in this area that chiropractic has experienced the greatest challenge to its legitimacy. Historical chiropractic has not developed a strong research paradigm, and the number of active scholars in the profession has been small. During the last decade, however, we have witnessed the exciting emergence of the chiropractic scholar. Although much remains to be accomplished, an essential prerequisite for this activity must be a systematization of the theories and research so far accumulated by chiropractic. This present work attempts a logical and orderly presentation of the theories and research and, therefore, not only will serve as a guide to this body of theory through our literature to those outside the profession but also, it is hoped, will provide a focus on the fundamental theoretical problems for those engaged in chiropractic research.

In the health field, care is best where research is best, and education is best when our students are exposed to both exemplary care and exemplary research and where they, in turn, can contribute to these processes. The present work should provide a challenge and a stimulus for chiropractors and students alike to

vii

become actively involved in the empirical research that will enhance the care of our patients.

I. D. COULTER, PhD
President
Canadian Memorial
Chiropractic College

May 30, 1985

Preface to the Second Edition

Less than a score of years ago, there was very little if any objective clinical chiropractic research on which a text such as this could focus. It is indeed exciting and gratifying to be able to report that in the last 5 years since the first edition of *The Chiropractic Theories*, significant advances have been made in several areas of chiropractic research. Chiropractic doctors have seen their research published in refereed medical and chiropractic journals and a medical textbook, and several chiropractic textbooks have been published by the medical publisher, Williams & Wilkins of Baltimore.

Medical cooperation with chiropractic doctors is apparently increasing, largely as a result of legal and economic conditions. Hence, one result of the Wilk et al. antitrust suit against the American Medical Association has been out-of-court settlements by several codefendants with the chiropractic plaintiffs. For example, in settling with the chiropractic plaintiffs the Board of Governors of the American Academy of Physical Medicine and Rehabilitaton stated (1), "It is the position of the American Academy of Physical Medicine and Rehabilitation that, except as provided by law . . . [,] there is and should be no ethical or collective impediment to full professional cooperation between chiropractors and medical physicians specializing in physical medicine and rehabilitation." Although it is unfortunate that cooperation between chiropractic and medicine has to be of the "shotgun wedding" variety, it will, nevertheless, be to the advantage of our patients that dialogue and research have begun.

In an effort to bring forward recent advances in chiropractic research, this text has been updated, expanded, and revised. Dr. Reed B. Phillips has contributed the chapter entitled, "Development of Theory." This chapter has met a need in this book for discussion of the principles of theory as well as for understanding the difference between theory and hypothesis. Several new illustrations in the text should highlight complicated concepts and make them more understandable. A significant amount of new information has been added to several chapters, notably those involving neurodystrophic phenomena, correction of the subluxation, and the cord compression hypothesis. It is hoped that these additions have made the text more readable.

We cannot conclude that we have all the answers, and in fact we are only now beginning to uncover some of the answers that have plagued chiropractic since its inception. If a lack of objective clinical research was the enigma of the profession, however, an abundance of clinical trials should soon provide a new cornerstone. Until that time we must agree with our medical counterparts in England who stated (2):

> Until there is a greater knowledge of spinal pathology, we are prepared to leave unsolved the enigmas of why and how spinal manipulation works. We are quite content to go on using an empirical remedy.

ROBERT A. LEACH, DC, FICC
March 1, 1985

References

1. Board of Governors: Professional association with chiropractors. *Arch Phys Med Rehabil* 62:1–4, 1981.
2. Ebbetts J: The present position of manipulative medicine. *Practitioner* 222:798–801, 1979.

Preface to the First Edition

The quest for truth rarely brings knowledgeable men and women to the same conclusion early in the search. Sometimes old theories are replaced by newer ones which are tried, tested, and used but still may fail. In other instances the newer theories may be rejected through debate instead of objective scientific experimentation. I believe the latter has been the case with chiropractic theories. From the evidence I will bring forth in this monograph I would hope that at the very least, men and women of science—who may have previously sought to avoid controversy—would demand more research in this field.

It would be great if science could document and explain all life processes and the pathogenesis of all diseases *today*; then health practitioners of the various healing arts would merely sit down together and decide the most obvious course of treatment for their patients. However, seldom in life is the most ideal course taken, and certainly science has yet to uncover even some of the fundamental causes of bodily function in health and disease. So instead humans have passed down through the ages methods for treating the various ailments that are sometimes, at best, ridiculous. As recently as several hundred years ago, one method of treating backache was to strap the unsuspecting patient onto a ladder which was then dropped off a rooftop (1). Archaic as that may sound, some of our modern-day practices may not always offer better results. That is not to say that our modern-day orthopedic, neurologic, and osteopathic methods are without good result. But time and time again the patient who has suffered through the good intent of several doctors will finally make his or her way to the so-called "quack" down the street, and several simple adjustments will result in relief of the complaint.

Much of this relief can be ascribed to the psychosomatic theory. However, detailed scientific study has already revealed several somewhat astonishing facts. Researchers at the University of Colorado (UofC) have already shown that the dorsal spinal nerve roots are extremely susceptible to compression in comparison with the peripheral nerve trunks (2). These and similar findings should stimulate more research. Yet in 1975 one major consumer magazine not only ignored the UofC research—in two articles on chiropractic—but went on to emphasize the conclusions of other scientists who have come to unacceptable and unobjective conclusions (see Chapter 6) (3-5). Such reporting undermines the search for truth and inhibits the right of the patient to seek that care which will prove most beneficial. As a former student of journalism I am still amazed that a reputable journal took such a slant, but at last something positive has come of it all. This book. In it I have endeavored to show that many authorities in the fields of science and medicine have already contributed to chiropractic theories with clinical, experimental, and postmortem studies and observations.

In the past, medical doctors would generally refrain from usage of the word "subluxation," but now it appears to have become nearly colloquial. In a book released recently, Helfat and Gruebel-Lee (6) refer to intervertebral and rotational subluxation as well as subluxation of the symphysis pubis! These orthopedic surgeons even refer to manipulation in the reduction of subluxations. Jackson (7), Hadley (8) and others in the medical field have contributed recently to this new wave of thought. They speak freely of the effects of subluxations in their literature. From direct spinal cord pressure (see Chapter 7) to vertebral artery insufficiency (see Chapter 9) to nerve root irritation or compression (see Chapter 6), these medical doctors have implicated the subluxation as a possible etiology.

Such acceptance is at first received with great relief, but the voice in the shadow tells us to be careful; medical research, with its massive funding and integration, could easily be cranked up with visions of supporting the medical specialist in manipulation instead of the chiropractor. This raises a fundamental question that is asked time and time again, "Should chiropractic be ushered into the fold of medicine?" We in chiropractic believe that the natural approach to health is the rational approach, and that—excepting the more severe cases—more aggressive treatment should be the last resort, not the first. In contrast, the medical approach to health is largely drug and surgery oriented; there is little consideration given to building the body's inherent recuperative powers by natural means. This represents a fundamental difference between chiropractic and medical science and is the major reason why I believe both should remain independent. This mandates that chiropractic research be initiated on a broad scale to lead the profession in achieving and documenting positive results.

It hurts to know that as a profession we are still lagging in many areas. Research is clearly one of these areas. Early pioneers in chiropractic would often develop bold explanations for the phenomenal symptomatic results that they sometimes obtained utilizing chiropractic adjustive (specific manipulation) techniques (9, 10). However, most often these explanations were based upon inadequate information, and it is now outdated as well. These explanations were often then used to "justify" the use of chiropractic for the clinical treatment of one disease or another. Today there is an outcry among chiropractic practitioners as well as academicians, lawmakers, and scientists for clinical research that will provide concrete answers to the complicated question of "scope of practice" for chiropractors. While this book provides hypotheses to explain the excellent results chiropractors sometimes obtain in patients with varied disorders, based upon current scientific and medical literature, we do not imply that the hypotheses can justify the use of any clinical procedure. Only proper clinical research can justify the use of clinical procedures, including chiropractic adjustments. This is just as true for the procedure that is used to treat disease as it is for the procedure that is used for the "correction of the cause of dis-ease." In either case the procedure must be clinically shown to be effective; this must be done before the public can appreciate the full significance of chiropractic care.

The door of research is finally opening for the chiropractic profession. We must encourage and nurture it with our time, efforts, and the efforts of other scientists and independently qualified investigators. This is the only guarantee we have that chiropractic will remain a separate and distinct science. Interprofessional cooperation is still obviously of great importance, but intraprofessional research will focus on the needs of the doctor of chiropractic. Our techniques, analyses and theories can now begin to fall under the close scrutiny of scientists. In this way society will know the full significance of the chiropractic theories, methods, and results. I believe we would all be satisfied with the truth if we could only see it. In the meantime. we need never worry about truth slipping away, for as we all know, *nunquam perit veritas* (truth never perishes).

ROBERT A. LEACH, DC
Fall, 1979

References

1. Lomax E: Manipulative therapy: a historical perspective from ancient times to the modern era. In Goldstein M (ed): *The Research Status of Spinal Manipulative Therapy.* Washington, DC, Government Printing Office, 1975, pp 11–17.
2. Suh CH: Researching the fundamentals of chiropractic. In Suh CH (ed): *Proceedings of the 5th Annual Biomechanics Conference on the Spine.* Boulder, CO University of Colorado, 1974, pp 1–52.
3. Botta JR (ed): Chiropractors healers or quacks? Part 1: the 80-year war with science. *Consumer Rep* 40:542–547, 1975.
4. Botta JR (ed): Chiropractors healers or quacks? Part 2: how chiropractors can help— or harm. *Consumer Rep* 40:606–610, 1975.
5. Crelin ES: A scientific test of the chiropractic theory. *Am Sci* 61:574–580, 1973.
6. Helfet AJ, Gruebel-Lee DM: *Disorders of the Lumbar Spine.* Philadelphia, Lippincott, 1978.
7. Jackson R: *The Cervical Syndrome.* Springfield, IL, Charles C Thomas, 1978.
8. Hadley LA: *Anatomico-Roentgenographic Studies of the Spine.* Springfield, IL, Charles C Thomas, 1964.
9. Palmer DD: *The Science, Art and Philosophy of Chiropractic.* Portland, OR, Portland Printing House, 1910.
10. Palmer BJ: *The Subluxation Specific—The Adjustment Specific.* Davenport, IA, Palmer School of Chiropractic, 1934.

Acknowledgments

As this work goes into its second edition, the list of those whose efforts have made it possible continues to grow. To those whose constructive criticism made the first edition possible, Thomas D. S. Key, EdD, ScD, Mario A. Vitelli, PhD, DC, and R. J. Watkins, DC, DABCR, I again extend my heartfelt thanks.

To Robert Fritzius, BS, thanks for the illustrations and proof-reading help. You have been a real asset.

To those doctors who sent suggestions and comments to me regarding the first edition, I am truly grateful.

To Thomas Blackshear, BS, MS, your constructive criticism of the first edition was most helpful.

To Reed B. Phillips, DC, MSCM, DACBR, FICC, thank you for lending your expertise in development of theory to this text.

To Vicki, my appreciation for your preparation of the manuscript as well as for your ability to decipher the Williams & Wilkins Style Manual is indeed sincere.

To Williams & Wilkins, thank you for bringing your publishing expertise and quality to the chiropractic profession.

Finally and most importantly, I would like to thank God, the author and sustainer of life, for everything.

It were not best that we should
all think alike; it is difference
of opinion that makes horseraces.
Samuel Langhorne Clemens
(Mark Twain)

Contents

Section 1
Introduction

Section 2
Chiropractic Theories of
Subluxation Pathophysiology

Section 3
Validating Chiropractic Theories

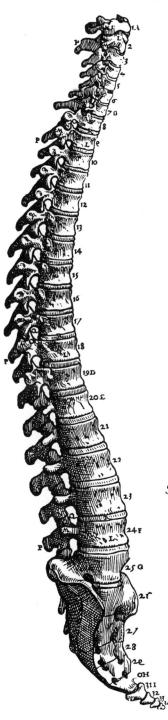

Section 1

Introduction

Men occasionally stumble over
the truth, but most of them
pick themselves up and hurry
off as if nothing had happened.

Sir Winston Leonard Spencer Churchill

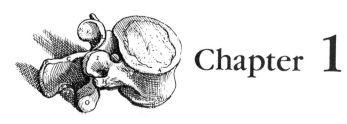

Chapter 1

General Introduction

For more than 90 years, chiropractors have enjoyed about the same friendly relations with medical doctors as Catholics have enjoyed with Protestants. It has been suggested that the reason for this animosity can be explained by differing interpretations of scientific data (1). This text has been written in order to provide the student, practitioner, and researcher with a comprehensive synopsis of scientific and medical literature relevant either directly or indirectly to chiropractic theories. Thus it is hoped that fact may be carefully sorted from fiction, and animosity may be wisely exchanged for understanding.

Many hypotheses have been developed regarding causes and effects of the intervertebral subluxation. Most of these hypotheses have been brought forward by one or more practitioners who then devised or patterned a technique after the hypothesis (Table 1.1). Certainly it is beyond the scope of this book to investigate them all; an attempt has been made, however, to present only those hypotheses that meet the following criteria: a) there is a substantial amount of scientific and/or medical literature in which the idea is either recognized or rejected, and b) based on these studies, there is a reasonable probability that the hypothesis is correct to some degree and therefore should be investigated further.

An understanding of the development of theory is necessary so that the reader is able to study the text and keep the data in proper perspective. Therefore, this second edition includes a new Chapter 2, "Development of Theory," written by Reed Phillips. Review of differences in terminology between the various health professions is the purpose of Chapter 3, "Manipulation Terminology in the Chiropractic, Osteopathic, and Medical Literature"; and the history of the various chiropractic hypotheses is explored briefly in Chapter 4.

Table 1.1.   Some principal chiropractic techniques in 1985

Technique	Inventor
Activator methods	W. C. Lee and A. W. Fuhr
Adjustment of the spastic muscle	Spastic Muscle Research Bureau, Inc.
Applied kinesiology	G. Goodheart
Atlas subluxation complex and correction	R. Gregory
Basic technique (Logan basic)	H. B. Logan
Bioenergetic synchronization	M. T. Morter
Chiroenergetics	E. H. Kimmel
Chiro-Manis treatment	J. M. Cox
Chiropractic neurobiochemical analysis	W. K. Ehmann
Concept therapy	H. Dill
Craniopathy	C. Cottam
Directional non-force technique	R. Van Rumpt
Endonasal and allied techniques	D. D. Gibbons
Fixation analysis-movement palpation	H. Gillet and M. Liekens
Gonstead technique	C. S. Gonstead
Gonstead cervical chair technique	C. S. Gonstead
Grostic procedure	J. Grostic
Kinesiology	F. Stoner
Life cervical technique	D. Jones
Mears technique	D. B. Mears
Palmer upper cervical	B. J. Palmer
Perianal postural reflex	R. J. Watkins
Pettibon method	B. E. Pettibon
Pierce-Stillwagon	W. V. Pierce
Polarity therapy	E. E. Jarvis
Receptor-tonus method	R. L. Nimmo
Reinert's disc move	O. C. Reinert
Rolfing	I. P. Rolf
Sacro-occipital technique	M. B. DeJarnette
Spears painless system	L. Spears and D. Spears
Spinal touch treatment	W. Lamar Rosquist
Thompson terminal point technique	J. C. Thompson
Toftness system	I. N. Toftness
Von Fox combination technique	R. Von Fox

Section 2 of this book contains chapters dealing with various chiropractic hypotheses, and Section 3 contains two chapters dealing specifically with chiropractic and manipulation research and research issues. An appendix includes information regarding pathologies that, with regard to symptomatology, may mimic biomechanical spinal lesions.

The axiom common to all chiropractic theories presented herein is that an intervertebral subluxation (subluxation is defined in Chapter 3) somehow alters the normal neurophysiological balance found in a healthy individual. It follows, therefore, that our primary hypothesis is that intervertebral subluxations occur with some frequency in the general population (see Chapter 5). From this there follow four important secondary hypotheses (Figure 1.1) which propose that in some cases this intervertebral subluxation may cause a) somatic afferent bombardment of the dorsal horn cells within the spinal cord, b) spinal cord compression, c) spinal nerve root compression, or d) vertebrobasilar arterial insufficiency in humans.

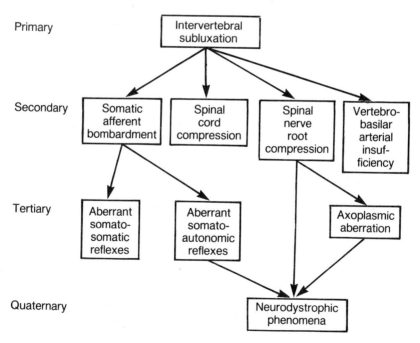

Figure 1.1. Hypothesized effects of intervertebral subluxation.

Likewise, there follow the tertiary hypotheses—dependent on verification of the validity of the secondary hypotheses—which propose that there are mechanisms by which aberrant somatosomatic reflexes, aberrant somatoautonomic reflexes, and axo plasmic aberration may occur. The principal quaternary hypothesis is that spinal nerve root compression, axoplasmic aberration, or aberrant somatoautonomic reflexes may contribute to neurodystrophic phenomena (see Chapter 12).

It should be noted that this author has, based on the available scientific literature, further developed these hypotheses. Working definitions have been adapted from the original authors' contributions in order to separate and classify the various hypotheses (Table 1.2). These may or may not coincide with the exact definitions given by the original authors as reported throughout this book. The definitions, however, reflect at least the principal idea of the hypotheses as originally presented.

In every instance, references from the medical and scientific literature are utilized to lend objectivity to the discussion. References by chiropractors are utilized mainly to verify the origin and topic of discussion within the chiropractic profession. Many of the references contained herein have not been readily available to the chiropractic profession, as years of dust have all but hidden them in the stacks at various medical and osteopathic college libraries. Unveiling these old data and comparing them with modern findings will, it is hoped, provide a clear overview of facts relevant to the various chiropractic theories.

Without a doubt, a clear presentation of chiropractic theories is needed. By official estimates, chiropractors treat 7.5 million patients yearly in the United States alone (2). Others have estimated that one quarter of the population of the United States has been to a chiropractor at one time or another, and that 86% of those patients believe that they have benefited from chiropractic care (3). In the 1970s, chiropractors saw official recognition of chiropractic colleges by the Office of Education of the Federal Department of Health, Education and Welfare, as well as inclusion of chiropractic services into Federal Medicare and Medicaid plans (1, 4). These political and social advances are impressive and suggest that equally impressive advances are needed in research of chiropractic theories. Before extensive research can begin however, a proper review of the literature is necessary. It is the

Table 1.2. Hypotheses pertaining to intervertebral subluxation[a]

Name	Statement of hypothesis
Intervertebral subluxation	Intervertebral subluxations are a common occurrence in the general population
Nerve compression	Intervertebral subluxations can interfere with the normal transmission of nerve energy (i.e., action potentials, etc.)
Cord compression	Intervertebral subluxations in some severe cases (and even in the absence of fracture/dislocation) may irritate or compress the spinal cord
Fixation	One type of subluxation is recognized by lessened mobility, soft-tissue involvement, aberrant neural reflexes, and segmental facilitation
Vertebrobasilar arterial insufficiency	Cervical intervertebral subluxations may cause deflection or compression of the vertebral arteries, which thereby gives rise to altered cerebral blood supply
Axoplasmic aberration	Axoplasmic flow may be altered when the spinal nerve roots become compressed or irritated by intervertebral subluxations
Somatoautonomic reflex	Somatic afferent bombardment of dorsal horn cells, which may result from spinal fixations, can alter normal autonomic reflexes
Neurodystrophic	Neural dysfunction is stressful to the visceral and other body structures, and this "lowered tissue resistance" can modify the nonspecific and specific immune responses and alter the trophic function of the involved nerves

[a] Adapted from sources cited in the various chapters.

purpose of this text to provide such a background which is necessary for research as well as for debate and future study.

The presentation of data in this book follows standard journal style. Following Chapter 4, chapters begin with a review of literature (chiropractic, medical, and/or scientific) dealing with the subject matter at hand. Reviews of clinical, experimental and, in some cases, postmortem studies are included in this discussion. A general discussion and a section on clinical applications of the data may precede the short summary, which acts to highlight important concepts. This format is designed to simplify the presentation of these studies, which might otherwise appear to be too complex for quick comprehension.

Outstanding research in biomechanics, neurophysiology, and neurochemistry at the University of Colorado is already providing answers to questions in basic chiropractic science (5–9). Studies at the various chiropractic colleges are supplying additional data of much significance clinically (see Chapter 13). These endeavors are clearly marking the onset of a new era for chiropractic science. It is within the scope of this book to review previous data in an effort to help guide future research as well as provide a better understanding of chiropractic theories for the practitioner and student.

References

1. Botta JR (ed): Chiropractors healers or quacks? Part 1: the 80-year war with science. *Consumer Rep* 40:542–547, 1975.
2. Howie LJ: Utilization of selected medical practitioners: United States, 1974. *Int Rev Chiropractic* 32:41–47, 1978.
3. Pollack JH: Do chiropractors really help you? *Ladies Home J* 89:91–92, 168, 1972.
4. Davidson GM (ed): US Dept of HEW issues approval, Council on Chiropractic Education is now the official accrediting agency for all colleges. *Dig Chiropractic Econ* 17:6, 1974.
5. Suh CH: Researching the fundamentals of chiropractic. In Suh CH (ed): *Proceedings of the 5th Annual Biomechanics Conference on the Spine.* Boulder, CO, University of Colorado, 1974, pp 26–45.
6. Sharpless SK: Susceptibility of spinal roots to compression block. In Goldstein M (ed): *The Research Status of Spinal Manipulative Therapy.* Washington, DC, Government Printing Office, 1975, pp 155–161.
7. Suh CH: The fundamentals of computer aided x-ray analysis of the spine. *J Biomech* 7:161–169, 1974.
8. Kelly PT: Mouse brain protein composition during postnatal development: an electrophoretic analysis. In Suh CH (ed): *Proceedings of the 6th Annual Biomechanics Conference on the Spine.* Boulder, CO, University of Colorado, 1975, pp 263–312.
9. Gerran RA, Groswald DE, Luttges MW: Triethyltin toxicity as a model for degenerative disorders. *Pharmicol Biochem Behav* 5:299–307, 1976.

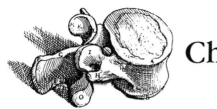

Chapter *2*

Development of Theory

*I*n the course of recorded history, the presence of chiropractic has been brief. To appreciate the material contained in this text, one must obtain a greater awareness of a) the historical development of knowledge, b) the composition of a theory, and c) the purpose of theory.

Historical Development of Knowledge

Common-sense thinking about life occurs even in the simplest of societies. Life is made up of incidents and encounters on which people reflect and from which people generalize. The lore or folk wisdom of a people is the essence of their "common sense" and helps to maintain social order.

There are things people do and things that happen to them that are not considered part of "everyday events." People have accidents or become ill and die. Such things tend to defy the explanatory formulas of folk wisdom.

In an effort to explain tragic, unexpected, and other frustrating events in life, mankind turned to magic and religion. The effects of magic on intellectual life were stifling. Rational analysis was not allowed. Religious institutions with powerful sanctions at their disposal were also very effective in obtaining intellectual conformity. Alternate explanations about human nature could result in excommunication.

Socrates, in the classical Greek period, is credited with the establishment of "rational proof" as a way to force all ideas to stand (or fall) on their own merit. Aristotle laid the foundations of logic; and others, such as Thales, Pythagoras, and Euclid established a practical application of mathematics (1).

Philosophy became the discipline of the West, and folk lore, magic, and religion were transformed into logically consistent wholes by philosophers. True science was not yet established, however, for science lives by the extension of empirical knowledge.

The task of establishing and explaining new facts and ascertaining their authenticity became the lot of historians rather than philosophers. According to Martindale (2),

> historical thought itself becomes fully possible only to the degree that objective secular knowledge of the actual world is possible and desirable. Historical thought appeared in the Greek world under the same general conditions that favored the discovery of the rational proof. Also, in a parallel fashion, it went into comparative decline in the Roman world, where rhetorical and patriotic motives were dominant. Its deepest eclipse occurred in the medieval world, where the historical forgery testified to the domination of didacticism and propaganda over objectivity.

The importance of history, i.e., requiring dependable data and a broad reporting of the facts, was revived through the periods of the Renaissance and Enlightenment.

The following is a paraphrase of Martindale's analogy of sociology (3):

> Like folk wisdom, *science* aspires to generalization about events; unlike folk wisdom, it seeks abstract knowledge not bound by the normative patterns of local time and place. Like religious thought, *science* aspires to abstract knowledge; unlike religious thought, it is neither metaphysically inclined or subordinate to sacred institutions. Like philosophy, *science* aspires to a body of knowledge resting on intrinsic rather than extrinsic standards of validity—a knowledge formed into logically consistent wholes; unlike philosophy, it is empirical rather than *ethical* (as in the case of traditional philosophy). Like history, *science* aspires to empirical knowledge of *events*; unlike history, it aspires to a knowledge of the general rather than the unique, for, when all is said and done, *science* is *an organization* of knowledge.

Science was parented by philosophy and history, but it differs from its parents in its endeavor to find a systematic procedure for extending empirical knowledge. The elevation of the experimental procedure to a position of prestige brought science to the forefront of the advancement of knowledge.

The utilization of the "experiment" for the advancement of knowledge progressed most rapidly in the natural sciences as a formal extension of such artisans as Leonardo da Vinci (1452–1519) and such scientists as Galileo (1564–1642).

Once experimentation was established as a method for exploring the physical world, it expanded into other spheres, which made science far more influential than ever before. Experimentation for the purpose of systematically extending empirical knowledge, however, implies the presence of some governing force or directive purpose attached to this experimentation. Otherwise, how does one determine what is to be done in an experiment and for what purpose? That thought process which binds together the advancement of knowledge and the development of science is theory.

Composition of Theory

Scientific knowledge is basically a system for description and explanation. It can be useful for a) forming classification systems, b) predicting future events, c) explaining past events, d) providing a sense of explanation about what causes events, and e) providing some potential for controlling events. Systematized scientific knowledge is usually referred to as *theory*.

The term theory is frequently misused to refer to concepts, prescribed behavior, or untested ideas (hypotheses). A theory should be supported by empirical data to be considered systematized scientific knowledge.

Scientific knowledge is basically a collection of abstract theoretical statements. There are three different concepts of how these statements should be organized so as to constitute a theory: a set of laws, an axiomatic form, and a causal process.

A Set of Laws

One approach is to accept as part of scientific knowledge only those statements that can be considered laws. A set of laws is then considered to be a theory. All laws are directly supported by empirical research, which means that all concepts used in laws must have operational definitions that allow their identification in concrete situations.

Theory in the form of a set of laws is useful for providing a typology, predictions, and explanations and allows the potential for control. A sense of understanding of the phenomena discussed, however, is often lacking. Also, the use of any unmeasurable concept or hypothetical construct is prohibited, since this form of theory requires precise operational definitions in concrete settings.

Axiomatic Form

The axiomatic form of theory construction is most commonly employed in the field of mathematics. It consists of a set of definitions, corollaries, and propositions derived from the axioms, all of which are interrelated. As with the set-of-laws concept of theory, statements in the axiomatic form of theory can be used to logically derive explanations and predictions and can also be used to classify events. It fails to provide a sense of understanding, however, since the logical notion of explanation is utilized with this form of theory.

The axiomatic form of theory does not require that all concepts be measurable. The number of interrelated statements required is less than that with the set-of-laws form and thus allows research to be more efficient. Also, axiomatic theory allows examination of all consequences of the assumptions made, due to the nature of their interrelatedness.

Causal Process

The causal process form of theory is an interrelated set of definitions and statements that describe causal processes. This form of theory is the only form that provides a sense of understanding of the phenomena discussed, in addition to the formulation of typologies and the provision of explanations and predictions. The major difficulty with this form of theory is the determination of when all steps in a causal linkage have been specified.

The three forms of general theory construction have been presented in a brief and simplified manner to provide the reader with an appreciation of that with which theories are composed. Much of the material contained within this text will fall short of the definitions and descriptions just provided, and the critic may well be justified in saying that much of what is espoused as "chiropractic theory" has not yet been adequately supported by valid objective data.

An appreciation of how well-developed theory advances scientific research should be gained from the last section of this chapter which deals with the purpose of theory. With this appreciation should come an understanding of why research in chiropractic has been slow to develop.

Purpose of Research

As folk lore has given way to scientific experimentation in the acquisition of knowledge, certain basic assumptions have been made. First, the world about us is more than what is in our minds. Second, the world can be known through a method or process that enables communication to occur about what one finds. Third, knowing is usually assumed to have some purpose beyond just "knowing," such as dealing with problems of survival (4).

Initially, observation and experience provided the data for development of beliefs. With time, knowledge obtained by observation and experience was systematized into logical patterns. Systematized knowledge set the stage for experimentation.

History will quickly reveal, however, that the development of knowledge was a difficult process. Kuhn (5) provides an excellent treatise on the advancement of knowledge from paradigm to paradigm by a process he labels "scientific revolutions." He points out that in the absence of any paradigm (a prevailing consensus about the nature of the world), fact-gathering is often a random activity that creates a morass of information that is unrelated and equally relevant. Without some theoretical and methodological belief system that permits selection, evaluation, and criticism of the collection of facts, the interpretation of phenomena will differ from individual to individual and from one particular instance to another.

Since the beginnings of chiropractic, prevailing paradigms have been externally provided by science and medicine. The conceptual development of chiropractic, generally, has represented an anomaly to such prevailing concepts as the "germ theory" as the cause of disease (5). This anomalous position of chiropractic (i.e., being established on the premise that bodily functions are closely influenced by structural relationships of body parts) prevented acceptance within the prevailing paradigm during the first half of the twentieth century. As a result of this exclusion, chiropractic has been only minimally successful in attracting the resources and intellectual maturity required for the advancement of its ideology.

Thus chiropractic, as a science lacking an adequate prevailing consensus (paradigm), has wandered about within the morass of random fact-finding and has been unable to formulate an adequate theoretical foundation supported by valid empirical data. Numerous hypotheses, discussed in the following pages, have been developed, but the presence of a prevailing "set of laws" or "axioms" or "causal descriptions" supported by empirical data and experimentation have been nonexistent.

Only in the very recent past, as the prevailing paradigm of medicine has begun to crumble under the weight of chronic diseases and drug-resistant microorganisms, has science taken an interest in the hypotheses espoused by chiropractors.

With this new emphasis, a new paradigm based on systematized scientific knowledge formulated under experimental scrutiny will be formed. This paradigm may full well encompass the structural and the functional relationships of the body as part of the concept of health.

The challenge of the future for science generally and for chiropractic specifically is to define the paradigm and develop the theoretical basis that will provide the guidance for seeking empirical data. No longer can resources be expended on random fact-finding. The justification for the existence of a profession and a portion of the health of mankind is dependent on how well the challenge is met.

In the words of Karl Popper, "theories are the nets cast to catch what we call 'the world'; to rationalize, to explain, and to master it. We endeavour to make the mesh ever finer and finer."

References

1. Heath TL: *A History of Greek Mathematics.* Oxford, Clarendon Press, 1921, vol 1, p 145.
2. Martindale D: *The Nature and Types of Sociological Theory.* Boston, Houghton-Mifflin, 1960, pp 15–16.
3. Martindale D: *The Nature and Types of Sociological Theory.* Boston, Houghton-Mifflin, 1960, p 19.
4. Herrick JE: *Theory Building for Basic Institutional Change.* San Francisco, Reed-Eterorich Research Associates, 1977, p 4.
5. Kuhn TS (ed): The structure of scientific revolutions. In: *International Encyclopedia of Unified Science.* Chicago, University of Chicago Press, 1970.

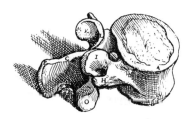

Chapter *3*

Manipulation Terminology in the Chiropractic, Osteopathic, and Medical Literature

*T*hree major healing professions, as well as other minor healing arts, utilize manipulation. Under the auspices of orthodox medicine, physical therapists and some medical doctors practice *manipulation*, "the forceful passive movement of a joint beyond its active limit of motion" (1). This technique involves the use of long levers and slow passive articular movements (2). In contrast, osteopathic manipulative therapy often involves active participation of the patient; the osteopathic profession uses a wide variety of manipulative and mobilization techniques (3). The chiropractic profession is the largest health profession in the world in which intervertebral manipulation is the central method of treatment. Chiropractic manipulation is unique in many aspects, however. Chiropractic manipulation is called *adjustment* and involves the utilization of short-lever, specific, high-velocity, controlled forceful thrusts by hand or instrument which are directed at specific articulations (4). Although the actual techniques of chiropractic adjustment differ fundamentally from those of any other form of manipulation, the most significant difference lies in the theories behind its application.

Defining the Subluxation

Most health practitioners agree that the term "subluxation" is too vague (5–8). Yet it is perhaps the most widely used noun in chiropractic today; almost all chiropractic theory is based on the existence of subluxation. Experts in the fields of roentgenology and orthopedics hold differing opinions as to the characteristics and, hence, definition of intervertebral subluxation. Original definitions of the term centered around the static nature of many subluxations:

An incomplete or partial dislocation [(9)].

Semiluxation; an incomplete luxation or dislocation; though a relationship is altered, contact between joint surfaces remains [(10)].

A partial or incomplete separation; one in which the articulating surfaces remain in partial contact [(11)].

One of the earliest definitions, however, which was stated by Hieronymus in 1746 according to Watkins (7), includes the criterion of motion:

Subluxation of joints is recognized by lessened motion of the joints, by slight change in the position of the articulating bones and by pain[;] ...most displacements of vertebrae are subluxations rather than luxations.

The chiropractic pioneer and developer B. J. Palmer defined four criteria that the chiropractic profession could utilize to differentiate simple intervertebral misalignments from intervertebral subluxation. These criteria are a) misalignment of a vertebra in relationship to the ones above and below, b) occlusion of a foramen, c) pressure on nerves, and d) interference with the transmission of neural impulses (12). This was one of the early chiropractic definitions, and it implied that from the profession's point of view, misalignments became subluxations when interference with the nervous system occurred.

Modern chiropractic definitions combine Palmer's criteria of misalignment and neurological interference with Hieronymus' and, more recently, Junghanns' concepts of alteration of normal mobility of the joint; in addition to lessened joint mobility, however, increased mobility is now included in the definition of subluxation (13, 14). Perhaps the most acknowledged definition in chiropractic today was presented at the National Institutes for Neurological Diseases and Stroke (now the National Institute of

Neurological and Communicative Disorders and Stroke, NINCDS)
workshop on spinal manipulative therapy (15):

> A subluxation is the alternation of the normal dynamics, anatomical
> or physiological relationships of contiguous articular structures.

This definition is broad enough that it may be applied to most
modern chiropractic theories and certainly to those theories presented in this text. Therefore, as Suh (16) points out, the chiropractic definition implies that neurophysiological and biomechanical abnormalities give the subluxation "a living character." By this
definition, neither cadaver studies nor static roentgenographs
would by sufficient to verify fully or to reject the existence of a
subluxation. This makes the study and research of the subluxation
very difficult.

The work of Illi (17), Watkins (7), Howe (18), and others in
the field of chiropractic roentgenology was used to devise a
specific subluxation terminology such as that set forth in the *Basic
Chiropractic Procedural Manual* (19) (Table 3.1). This new
terminology takes into account the many variables that may occur
in any given subluxation. For example, from the x-ray the chiropractor may note a combination static subluxation including both
lateral flexion malposition and rotational malposition; or, on
motion palpation and a flexion-extension radiographic series, the
doctor may note hypermobility or aberrant motion. Thus, modern
terminology in chiropractic allows the doctor to describe the
parameters of each subluxation more specifically than was previously possible.

Chiropractic roentgenologists such as MacRae (20) have determined the various criteria for intervertebral subluxations according to radiographic data. For example, atlas subluxation (according to radiographic criteria only) may be determined by the
method of Bull, atlantodental interval (ADI), digastric line, roentgenographic upper cervical alignment, horizontal line of atlas,
George's line, and periodontal space (20). Radiographic criteria
for thoracic, lumbar, and pelvic subluxation have also been determined.

Hildebrandt (21) prefers the term *spinal dysarthria* to intervertebral subluxation and suggests that this term implies both static
and functional aspects of the lesion. He describes a classification
system for spinal dysarthrias which includes the following:

Table 3.1. Categories of spinal and paraspinal subluxations[a]

A. Static intersegmental subluxations
  1. Flexion malposition
  2. Extension malposition
  3. Lateral flexion malposition
  4. Rotational malposition
  5. Anterolisthesis (spondylolisthesis)
  6. Retrolisthesis
  7. Laterolisthesis
  8. Altered interosseous spacing (decreased or increased)
  9. Osseous foraminal encroachments
B. Kinetic intersegmental subluxations
  1. Hypomobility (fixation subluxation)
  2. Hypermobility (loosened vertebral motor unit)
  3. Aberrant motion
C. Sectional subluxation
  1. Scoliosis and/or alterations of curves secondary to muscular imbalance
  2. Scoliosis and/or alterations of curves secondary to structural asymmetries
  3. Decompensation of adaptational curvatures
  4. Abnormalities of motion
D. Paravertebral subluxations
  1. Costovertebral and costotransverse disrelationships
  2. Sacroiliac subluxations

[a] From Inman OB: *Basic Chiropractic Procedural Manual*. Des Moines, American Chiropractic Association, 1973 (19). (Used by permission of the American Chiropractic Association.)

Type A—vertebral motor unit unable to move from normal resting position; fixed in normal alignment (etiologies: bilateral paraspinal muscle spasms, facet jamming, discopathy, pathologic ankylosis, etc.).

Type B—motor unit unable to move properly through its range of motion; partially fixed in or out of normal alignment (etiologies: unilateral muscle spasm, unilateral facet jamming, etc.).

Type C—vertebral motor unit unable to return to normal resting position; fixed outside normal alignment (etiologies: bilateral muscle spasm, facet jamming).

Haldeman (22) describes a manipulable spinal lesion as one having the following characteristics: vertebral malposition, abnormal vertebral motion, lack of joint play, palpable soft-tissue changes, and muscle contraction or imbalance. Faucret et al. (23)

describe 14 clinical signs of intervertebral subluxation. These efforts underscore the importance of further quantification and characterization of the intervertebral subluxation and the subsequent development of a terminology system even more descriptive than that which is now available.

Subluxation terminology of the future should become more definitive, in light of the mathematical distortion analysis research of Suh (16) at the University of Colorado. It has been known for many decades that due to the diverging nature of x-rays, radiographs are inherently distorted; the computer-aided distortion analysis recently devised will allow for measurement of intervertebral subluxations with nearly total accuracy (16, 24, 25). Studies based on highly accurate analyses, such as this new technique, will provide the profession with scientifically acceptable data concerning the true position of vertebral structures. Measurements could be standardized and the exact spinal configurations could then be transferred from chiropractor to chiropractor even in the absence of film. Until such progress is made, the definition of subluxation as reported to the NINCDS will suffice for this text; additional terminology as recorded in Table 3.1 will be utilized when necessary. Please note that for the purpose of discussion the hypomobile kinetic intersegmental subluxation will be hereafter designated a spinal fixation (SF) (see Chapter 8).

Approaches to Spinal Disorders and Terminology

Although it is not the design of this book to describe medical, orthopedic, neurologic, and osteopathic spinal lesions, treatments, and hypotheses, nevertheless, it will be helpful to briefly summarize their respective approaches to spinal disorders and terminology (Table 3.2).

Medical doctors who specialize in the preservation and restoration of the skeletal system and its articulations are known as orthopedists. Some members of the orthopedic as well as the neurologic community believe that subluxation occurs only with disc thinning or other similar degeneration of the functional unit (a *functional unit* is made up of an anterior segment, which consists of any two vertebral bodies separated by an intervertebral disc, and a posterior segment, which consists of the articular

Table 3.2.   Terminological differences among manipulators

Term	Chiropractic	Osteopathic	Medical
Treatment	Adjustment	Osteopathic manipulative therapy	Manipulation (manual therapy)
Disorder	Intervertebral subluxation	Somatic dys-function	Vertebral (spinal) lesion

facets) (26, 27). In general, it is safe to summarize that most experts in the orthopedic field acknowledge even frequent occurrence of subluxations but assume that these disorders play only a minor role in body dysfunction (see Chapters 6 and 8).

The branch of medicine which deals with the nervous system in health and disease is neurology. Neurologists generally focus their attention on pathological disorders of the nervous system. The famous *Handbook of Clinical Neurology*—which is anything but a handbook—is composed of many volumes and many thousands of pages which describe the pathologies and disorders studied by neurologists. The following definition of subluxation is taken from the *Handbook of Clinical Neurology* (5):

> A subluxation is a somewhat vague but nevertheless commonly used expression which may be defined as a partial disruption of the articular surfaces.

Although Guttmann (28) reports that subluxation in the cervical spine may cause rotation and/or tilt of the head, other neurologists, such as Braakman and Penning (29), believe that a diagnosis of subluxation in the cervical spine is a mistake. Braakman and Penning apparently prefer the terms "cervical sprain" and "hyperanteflexion sprain." It is noteworthy that they use "hyperanteflexion sprain" as another term for "anterior subluxation." Braakman and Penning believe that conservative management for children with hyperanteflexion sprain of the second and third cervical vertebrae (i.e., a Minerva jacket or collar and prolonged bed rest) is not effective on a short-term basis. They note that, with time, children generally get better regardless of the treatment utilized. In adults with hyperanteflexion sprain, however, management is different (29):

> In adults[,] surgical fusion may be indicated in cases of recurrent or severe angulation. In minor angulation a policy of "wait and see" is

adopted. Fusion is effected by bone grafting either by the posterior [approach] or [by the] anterior approach. Wiring may help in establishing reduction of the angulation during the operation.

This treatment would be considered radical by the average chiropractor, who treats such cases by adjustment and other modalities when these are deemed necessary.

Other specialities in the medical field also deal with spinal complaints and disorders. In physical medicine, the doctor treats back pain patients with exercises and supports, when necessary, and utilizes medication and traction less often (30). Disc surgery is used as a last alternative and only when indicated. Cailliet (30) describes the conservative approach to low back pain which is used by the specialist in physical medicine:

> As established from the history and physical examination, the treatment of the mechanical low-back pain is based on the correction of faulty *static* posture and faulty *kinetic* mechanism of the lumbar spine.
> *Static* abnormalities are essentially the result of faulty posture, and correction of these faults with resultant good posture should result in a pain-free stance. Adequate flexibility, good muscle tone, and proper concept of good kinesthetics are essential for the maintenance of proper posture.

Probably most closely aligned to chiropractic, at least in theory, is the osteopathic profession. Osteopathy is based on Still's belief that the body is capable of making its own remedies against disease and other toxic conditions when the structural relationships are functioning properly, along with proper nutrition and favorable environmental conditions (31). The following is the modern definition of the *osteopathic spinal lesion*, also known as "somatic dysfunction," which in chiropractic is probably most analogous to subluxation (32):

> Impaired or altered function of related components of the somatic (body framework) system; skeletal, arthrodial, and myofascial structures, and related vascular, lymphatic, and neural elements.

Perhaps the majority of osteopaths give some thought to the somatic system when they are treating disease processes; the profession, however, seems to be moving away from this holistic view.

It appears that each branch of medicine has its own beliefs and theories to support sometimes-opposing concepts and therapies.

Probably the only agreement among the experts is that there can be no agreement on terms, treatment, and theories until more data and research are forthcoming. The situation was best described by Goldstein (15) who made the following comment at the previously mentioned spinal manipulative therapy workshop:

> The presentations on *x-ray examination* of the patient with a suspected "nidus" polarized discussion. Those utilizing x-ray examination for this purpose presented slides and quoted references attesting to the efficacy and safety of the diagnostic technique; others just as authoritatively presented slides and quoted references attesting to the inaccuracy and dangers of using the technique for this purpose.

Characterization and quantification of the intervertebral subluxation will allow members of all the healing arts to carry on a more meaningful dialogue regarding spinal manipulation and spinal lesions. Certainly in chiropractic this research goal has high priority and can only result in a better understanding of the effects of intervertebral subluxation.

References

1. Friel JP (ed): *Dorland's Illustrated Medical Dictionary*, ed 25. Philadelphia, Saunders, 1974, p 909.
2. DeHesse P: *Chirotherapy*. Prescott, AZ, published privately, 1946, pp 13–26.
3. Greenman PE: Manipulative therapy in relation to total health care. In Korr IM (ed): *The Neurobiologic Mechanisms in Manipulative Therapy*. New York, Plenum, 1978, pp 43–53.
4. Janse J: History of the development of chiropractic concepts; chiropractic terminology In Goldstein M (ed): *The Research Status of Spinal Manipulative Therapy*. Washington, DC, Government Printing Office, 1975, pp 25–42.
5. Braakman R, Penning L: Injuries to the cervical spine. In Vinken PJ, Bruyn GW (eds): *Handbook of Clinical Neurology*. Injuries to the spinal cord part 1. New York, Elsevier, 1976, vol 25, p 242.
6. Haldeman S: The pathophysiology of the spinal subluxation. In Goldstein M (ed): *The Research Status of Spinal Manipulative Therapy*. Washington, DC, Government Printing Office, 1975, pp 217–226.
8. Tower DB: Chairman's summary: evolution and development of the concepts of manipulative therapy. In Goldstein M (ed): *The Research Status of Spinal Manipulative Therapy*. Washington, DC, Government Printing Office, 1975, p 59.
9. Friel JP (ed): *Dorland's Illustrated Medical Dictionary*. ed 25. Philadelphia, Saunders, 1974, p 1488.
10. Hensyl WR (ed): *Stedman's Medical Dictionary*, ed 24. Baltimore, Williams & Wilkins, 1982, p 1356.
11. Palmer DD: *The Science, Art and Philosophy of Chiropractic*. Portland, OR, Portland Printing House, 1910, p 490.
12. Palmer BJ: *The Subluxation Specific—The Adjustment Specific*. Davenport, IA, Palmer School of Chiropractic, 1934, p 329.

13. Howe JW: The role of x-ray findings in structural diagnosis. In Goldstein M (ed): *The Research Status of Spinal Manipulative Therapy.* Washington, DC, Government Printing Office, 1975, pp 239-247.
14. Jackson R: *The Cervical Syndrome.* Springfield, IL, Charles C Thomas, 1978.
15. Goldstein M: Introduction, summary, and analysis. In Goldstein M (ed): *The Research Status of Spinal Manipulative Therapy.* Washington, DC, Government Printing Office, 1975, pp 3-7.
16. Suh CH: Computer-aided spinal biomechanics. In Haldeman S (ed): *Modern Developments in the Principles and Practice of Chiropractic.* New York, Appleton-Century-Crofts, 1980, pp 143-170.
17. Janse J: The concepts and research of Fred W. Illi. In Janse J (ed): *Principles and Practice of Chiropractic.* Lombard, IL, National College of Chiropractic, 1976, pp 51-70.
18. Howe JW: The chiropractic concept of subluxation and its roentgenological manifestations. *J Clin Chiropractic,* 64-70, September/October 1973.
19. Inman OB (ed): *Basic Chiropractic Procedural Manual.* Des Moines, American Chiropractic Association, 1973.
20. MacRae J: *Roentgenometrics in Chiropractic.* Toronto, published privately, 1974.
21. Hildebrandt RW: The scope of chiropractic as a clinical science and art: an introductory review of concepts. *J Manip Physiolog Ther* 1:7-17, 1978.
22. Haldeman S: Spinal manipulative therapy in the management of low back pain. In Finneson BE (ed): *Low Back Pain,* ed 2. Philadelphia, Lippincott, 1980, pp 245-275.
23. Faucret B, Mao W, Nakagawa T, Spurgin D, Tran T: Determination of bony subluxations by clinical, neurological and chiropractic procedures. *J Manip Physiolog Ther* 3:165-176, 1980.
24. Schram SB, Hosek RS: Error limitations in x-ray kinematics of the spine. *J Manip Physiolog Ther* 5:5-10, 1982.
25. Grostic J: Some observations on computer-aided x-ray analysis. *Int Rev Chiropractic* 33:38-41, 1979.
26. Sunderland S: The anatomy of the intervertebral foramen and the mechanisms of compression and stretch of nerve roots. In Haldeman S (ed): *Modern Developments in the Principles and Practice of Chiropractic.* New York, Appleton-Century-Crofts, 1980, pp 45-64.
27. Sandler B: Cervical spondylosis as a cause of spinal cord pathology. *Arch Phys Med Rehabil* 42:650-659, 1961.
28. Guttmann L: Conservative management. In Vinken PJ, Bruyn GW (eds): *Handbook of Clinical Neurology.* Injuries to the spinal cord part 2. New York, Elsevier, 1976, vol 26, pp 289-306.
29. Braakman R, Penning L: Injuries to the cervical spine. In Vinken PJ, Bruyn GW (eds): *Handbook of Clinical Neurology.* Injuries to the spinal cord part 1. New York, Elsevier, 1976, vol 25, pp 242, 341-345.
30. Cailliet R: *Low Back Pain Syndrome.* Philadelphia, Davis, 1968, p 77.
31. Wright HM: *Perspectives in Osteopathic Medicine.* Kirksville, MO, Kirksville College of Osteopathic Medicine, 1976.
32. Northup GW: History of the development of osteopathic terminology. In Goldstein M (ed): *The Research Status of Spinal Manipulative Therapy.* Washington, DC, Government Printing Office, 1975, pp 43-51.

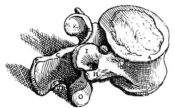

Chapter 4

History of the Chiropractic Theories

*I*n the Far East around 2700 B.C., Kong-Fou gave probably the first written account of manipulation, according to Dintenfass (1). It is known that ancient civilizations from Babylonia to Central America to Tibet practiced manipulative therapies (1). More interesting, however, is the possibility that Hippocrates used manipulation not only to reposition vertebrae but also thereby to cure a wide variety of dysfunctions (2). This may have been the first disease-oriented application of what is today known as spinal manipulation. For the next two thousand years, manipulation apparently was used only to correct luxations and other spinal complaints, but by the early nineteenth century new developments again focused attention on the spinal cord.

Spinal Irritation

Discoveries such as the Bell-Magendie law and Marshall Hall's theory of reflex action placed the spinal cord in the medical limelight. "Spinal irritation" became a clinical entity following coinage of the term by Thomas Brown in 1828 in the *Glasgow Medical Journal* (2, 3). In 1832, the *American Journal of Medical Sciences* began carrying news from Europe about spinal irritation, and eminent physicians reported diagnostic progress (2). There seemed to be no limit to what diseases spinal irriration could cause, and tenderness of the appropriate vertebra clinched the diagnosis. J. Evans Riadore, who wrote *Irritation of the Spinal Nerves* in 1843, is probably the contemporary father of the nerve compression hypothesis according to Donald Tower (4), the former director of the National Institutes for Neurological and

Communicable Diseases and Stroke. Tower states that Riadore, a physician, had written, ". . . if any organ is deficiently supplied with nervous energy or of blood, its functions immediately, and sooner or later its structure, become deranged . . . ." Apparently Riadore concluded that irritation of the spinal nerve roots resulted in diseases; he even advised manipulation to treat this disorder. It is noteworthy that Riadore made these conclusions 2 years before D. D. Palmer, the founder of chiropractic, was even born (5). In 1894, Sir William Gowers (3), a prominent physician in the London Hospital, said, "function depends upon the release of force—nerve force." Thus, the stage was set for Andrew Taylor Still (the founder of osteopathy) and D. D. Palmer. Still and Palmer were probably outraged at the late-nineteenth-century medical treatment for spinal irritation, which included cauterization and application of leeches to the tender dorsal area (2). It is probable then that the hypothesis adopted by Palmer was largely a result of this nineteenth-century contemporary medical thought and that manipulation was adopted as a more conservative mode of treatment than the aforementioned remedies.

Palmer's Contribution

D. D. Palmer (5) founded chiropractic in 1895 in Iowa. He admitted several times that he was not the first to utilize manipulation for the correction of human ailments, but he did claim to be the first to utilize the spinous and transverse processes of vertebrae as levers enabling the doctor to "rack" the bones back to their normal juxtaposition. Palmer (5) also "named the mental act of accumulating knowledge, the cumulative function, corresponding to the physical vegetative function—growth of intellectual and physical—together, with the science, art and philosophy—chiropractic." Palmer's writings are a classic to the profession today. His textbook, *The Science, Art and Philosophy of Chiropractic*, included some contradictions in terminology. (For example, on page 295 Palmer reviews an article and then states, "Narrowing of intervertebral foramina might squeeze, pinch or compress the outgoing nerves, but impinge upon them never." On page 70, however, he concludes, "A bone does not pinch upon a nerve. The condition of pressure upon a nerve is known as an impingement.") Nevertheless, the point of the text rang true and led chiropractic forward to take its place as the second largest health profession in the world. Palmer described in great detail the entire impingement process and its effects, according to his knowledge at that time. He recognized various causes of disease, such as accidents and poisons, but rejected the *germ* theory as well as the *humoral* theory of disease causation (i.e., that disease results when the four humors—blood, phlegm, and yellow and black bile—are imbalanced). Instead, Palmer proposed that sub-luxations cause increased or decreased body *tonus* and that this is disease. Thus to Palmer in 1910, accidents and poisons resulted in subluxations which caused nerve impingement and thereby disease. Correction of the spinal subluxation was followed by convalescence and a return to optimum health. This was the beginning of what are today known as the nerve compression and neurodystrophic hypotheses (see Chapters 6 and 12).

In 1912, Gregory (3) reiterated Palmer's thesis and explained:

> The most frequent point of mechanical interference with the normal nerve function is where the nerves make their exit from the neural canal through the foramina formed by notches in the adjacent pedicles of vertebrae.

Gregory, a medical doctor and student of Palmer, published a complex treatise, *Spinal Treatment Science and Technique,* in which he stated that excitability, conductivity, reflexivity, and efferent transmission may all be affected by nerve interference.

In 1921, Carver (6) published the famous *Carver's Chiropractic Analysis.* Carver differed little from Palmer in his interpretation of the nerve impingement theory.

Turner's book, *The Rise of Chiropractic* (7), published in 1931, seems to be based on much information that is probably not even available today. He states that Palmer disclaimed credit for theories supporting chiropractic in several of his writings. He claimed that Palmer's great contribution was invention of the science of replacing vertebrae by utilizing vertebral processes as levers.

Goldthwait (8), a famous orthopedist, in 1934 stated:

> There is, however, another type of nerve root irritation showing similar pathology and functional disturbance due to mechanical causes, usually the result of pressure or stretching of the nerve roots.

Goldthwait was perhaps the first of the modern medical scientists to step forward in acknowledgment of the existence of nerve root compression and irritation. Yet as is amply pointed out in the succeeding chapters, a host of medical and scientific investigators have since studied nerve root compression. In all fairness, however, Goldthwait did not accept the idea that such compression could cause disease. Instead, he proposed that nerve irritation or compression at the root caused only referred pain which only mimicked visceral disease and did not actually cause it. Thus, Goldthwait reasoned, by correction of the spinal lesion the symptoms disappeared and the patient believed disease had been cured. The phenomenon of referred pain by this mechanism has since been documented (see Chapters 6 and 11), but other mechanisms have also been described (axoplasmic damming, nerve root compression resulting in spinal cord ischemia, etc.), which suggests that Goldthwait had taken a narrow viewpoint (see Chapters 8, 9 and 10).

Throughout the 1930s, important research in Europe and in Russia—under the leadership of Speransky (9)—shed new light on the implications of damage to the nervous system. In America, Kuntz (10) and others conducted research along similar lines of thought (see Chapter 12).

Hole-in-One Technique

B. J. Palmer, D. D. Palmer's son, extended the nerve impingment theory. In his *The Science of Chiropractic*, he said (11),

> . . . subluxations, which would diminish the size of lateral foramina[,] would, by the fact of subluxation of bone on bone, diminish the size of the opening from above downward on that spinal cord (without fracture or death), consequently this opens up a larger and broader viewpoint.

In essence, Palmer implied that not only nerve roots but also the cord itself could be damaged in cases of subluxation (see Chapter 7).

Palmer (12) established four criteria for his definition of "subluxation": misalignment of the vertebra in relation to adjacent segments, occlusion of a foramen (including the spinal canal and the intervertebral foramina) that contains nerves, pressure upon nerves, "and interference to transmission of mental impulse supply" (i.e., action potentials). Palmer went on to assert, however, that the only two vertebrae in the spine which could be subluxated were the atlas and the axis (he predicted that it was only at these levels that "occlusion of a foramen" could result in spinal cord or nerve pressure from a subluxation; he incorrectly predicted that spinal nerve root compression could occur also at these levels but nowhere else in the spine). This hypothesis resulted in his formation of a chiropractic adjustive technique in which only the first or second cervical vertebrae were adjusted. Because this was the so-called "major" subluxation, Palmer's method of correction was called the "hole in one" (HIO) technique. It was Palmer's assertion that "no chiropractor can practice chiropractic without an NCM (neurocalometer)" and that any chiropractor not using the NCM with the HIO technique was incapable of practicing honestly, which led to the great division in the chiropractic profession (13). After he had delivered his talk entitled, "The Hour Has Struck," at the lyceum of the Palmer School of Chiropractic in 1924, only a small segment of the chiropractic profession would hold to his rigid beliefs (13). This author speculates that probably less than 5% of the profession still adheres to this technique today, to the exclusion of all other hypotheses and techniques.

Fixation Concept

Although experimental and clinical data were assembled regarding the nerve compression and cord compression hypotheses of the Palmers', the past few decades have marked the rise of yet another hypothesis which is based on the vertebral motor unit concept of Junghanns (14). Lack of proper motion, according to Junghanns' concept of joint motion, became one category for intervertebral subluxation (14). Originally reported in the medical and, later, the osteopathic literature, this concept was further promoted and expanded by Verner, Hviid, Homewood, and others in the chiropractic profession (R. J. Watkins, personal communication; and References 15–17). Especially significant is the idea that many subluxations are actually "fixations" in which the vertebrae are locked within their normal range of motion (see Chapter 8). According to this hypothesis, these spinal fixations can give rise to abnormal somatoautonomic as well as somatosomatic reflexes, by bombarding dorsal horn cells with afferent impulses. The somatoautonomic reflex hypothesis is the topic of Chapter 11. It is probable that to some degree such aberrant reflex activity could give rise to the neurodystrophic phenomena discussed in Chapter 12. Hence, the fixation concept is significant because it explains the genesis of a wide range of aberrant neural activity which has manifestations in the endocrine and immune systems also.

New-Age Progress

By the 1950s, a new era of scientific progress was beginning for the chiropractic profession. This was established by chiropractors such as B. J. Palmer (12, 18) whose extensive studies were designed to establish the difference between the normal nervous mechanism and the aberrant one. Palmer utilized every tool imaginable to measure nervous energy and the effects of subluxations. He used such machines as the Ellis Micro-Dynameter, the neurocalometer, neurotempometer, and the electroencephalo-neuromentimpograph (18, 19). Research data (18) were published which showed that his studies included hematological, basal metabolic, electrocardiographic, and many other tests to record changes under "controlled specific chiropractic care."

Although he was the major chiropractic researcher of the 1950s, he was not the only one. For chiropractic theories, there was Verner's, *The Science and Logic of Chiropractic* (20), which was as thorough and investigative as it was honest. At last, here was a chiropractor who was beginning to accept the role that germs play in disease, while he was redefining the role of the nervous system which not only fights disease processes (see Chapter 12) but also maintains the chemical and environmental control necessary for health (20):

> It should not be assumed that because the nervous system occupies such a supremely powerful or influential position, . . . the body can meet every emergency. It cannot. However, neural machanisms are always involved in infection and immunity, just as they are in everything else. Very frequently they dominate the situation; they hold the balance of power. It is in such cases that Chiropractic operating through such neural mechanisms, may be employed to advantage.

In 1953, Verner (21) teamed up with Weiant and Watkins to write *Rational Bacteriology.* In this book, they summarized the problem of dogmatic adherence to one theory or another:

> Some of the chiropractors have philosophically ignored bacteria as though they were non-existent. Others have theorized that bacteria

are scavengers. They have compared the "germ theory" ideology to that of flies as the cause of the manure pile. . . .

Chiropractors can now rise above the confusion of bacteriology and properly evaluate that science, instead of disregarding it, as few have done.

One of the monumental articles of this era was written by Hadley (22), a physician and roentgenologist. His studies not only verified the chiropractic position on subluxation, to some degree, but also went on to describe histologically the injured nerve roots that were compressed following a subluxation. Hadley's studies were of monumental importance to the chiropractic and spinal manipulation fields, for at last chiropractors had the raw data to help substantiate the nerve compression hypothesis. The age of unquestioned doubt was nearing its end; chiropractors and scientists had established to some degree what had once been only philosophical theory.

Scientific Revolution

By the late 1960s, the real scientific revolution had begun for chiropractic. Beginning in 1970 at the University of Colorado at Boulder, a series of biomechanics conferences were held (23). These conferences have continued under the direction of C. H. Suh; a computer model of the spine has been developed and at least one astonishing fact (the susceptibility of nerve roots to compression, which is discussed in Chapter 6) directly related to the nerve compression hypothesis has been uncovered. In addition, this government- and chiropractic-sponsored research effort has yielded new hypotheses also. For example, Luttges et al. (24) and Triano and Luttges (25) have demonstrated that compression or irritation or section of spinal nerves in test animals can alter their protein composition distal as well as proximal to the site of the site of injury (see Chapter 10). Because this research was partially supported by the chiropractic profession, we must conclude that these scientists have given us a new hypothesis which we will call the axoplasmic aberration hypothesis.

Another more recent hypothesis concerns cerebral blood flow and its regulation. Some chiropractors have noted that cervical intervertebral subluxations may compromise the arterial flow within the vertebral arteries (26–28). Since these arteries are a major source of the cerebral arterial system, it has been suggested, some symptoms in the cranium may be caused by disruption of the flow of these vessels.

Meanwhile, for the first time, chiropractic care has been studied by independent observers to determine its efficacy for children with learning disabilities and for adults with various back sprain and strain problems. In both groups, the results of care rendered by a chiropractor were compared with the results of care rendered by a physician (see Chapter 13).

These clinical data are the culmination of a new wave of attention which has been focused on chiropractic in recent years. One highlight of this attention has been the spinal workshops held recently at the National Institutes of Health and elsewhere (29–32). Participants in these workshops have included eminent physicians, osteopaths, chiropractors, and scientists. Several reports given at these conferences have been favorable to the various chiropractic theories. Even now (1985), however, chiropractic theories lack the broad experimental as well as clinical data which would bring them scientific credibility.

References

1. Dintenfass J: *Chiropractic: A Modern Way to Health.* New York, Pyramid, 1970.
2. Lomax E: Manipulative therapy: a historical perspective from ancient times to the modern era. In Goldstein M (ed): *The Research Status of Spinal Manipulative Therapy.* Washington, DC, Government Printing Office, 1975, pp 11–17.
3. Gregory A: *Spinal Treatment Science and Technique.* Oklahoma City, Palmer-Gregory College, 1912.
4. Tower D: Chairman's summary: evolution and development of the concepts of manipulative therapy. In Goldstein M (ed): *The Research Status of Spinal Manipulative Therapy.* Washington, DC, Government Printing Office, 1975, p 59.
5. Palmer DD: *The Science, Art and Philosophy of Chiropractic.* Portland, OR, Portland Printing House, 1910.
6. Carver W: *Carver's Chiropractic Analysis.* Oklahoma City, Carver Chiropractic College, 1921.
7. Turner C: *The Rise of Chiropractic.* Los Angeles, Powell, 1931.
8. Goldthwait JE: *Body Mechanics.* Philadelphia, Lippincott, 1934.
9. Speransky AD: *A Basis for the Theory of Medicine.* Leningrad, International, 1943.
10. Kuntz A: *The Autonomic Nervous System.* Philadelphia, Lea & Febiger, 1945.
11. Palmer BJ: *The Science of Chiropractic.* Davenport, IA, Palmer School of Chiropractic, 1911.
12. Palmer BJ: *The Subluxation Specific—The Adjustment Specific.* Davenport, IA, Palmer School of Chiropractic, 1934.
13. Gibbons RW: The evolution of chiropractic: medical and social protest in America. In Haldeman S (ed): *Modern Developments in the Principles and Practice of Chiropractic.* New York, Appleton-Century-Crofts, 1980, pp 3–24.
14. Schmorl G, Junghanns J: *The Human Spine in Health and Disease.* New York, Grune & Stratton, 1971.

15. Burns L (ed): Evidence of the existence of lesions. In Burns L (ed): *The Effects of Lumbar Lesions.* Chicago, Still Research Institute, 1917, pp 14–15.

16. Hviid H: A consideration of contemporary chiropractic theory. *J Natl Chiropractic Assoc* 25:17–18, 1955.

17. Homewood AE: *The Neurodynamics of the Vertebral Subluxation,* ed 3. St Petersburg, FL, Valkyrie Press, 1979.

18. Palmer BJ: *Chiropractic Clinical Controlled Research.* Davenport, IA, Palmer School of Chiropractic, 1951.

19. Maynard JE: *Healing Hands: The Story of the Palmer Family, Discoverers and Developers of Chiropractic.* Mobile, AL, Jonorm, 1977.

20. Verner JR: *The Science and Logic of Chiropractic.* Brooklyn, Cerasoli, 1941, p 220.

21. Verner JR, Weiant CW, Watkins RJ: *Rational Bacteriology.* New York, Wolf, 1953, p 204.

22. Hadley LA: Intervertebral joint subluxation, bony impingement and foramen encroachment with nerve root change. *Am J Roentgenol Rad Ther* 65:377–402, 1951.

23. Suh CH: Researching the fundamentals of chiropractic. In Suh CH (ed): *Proceedings of the 5th Annual Biomechanics Conference on the Spine.* Boulder, CO, University of Colorado, 1974, pp 1–52.

24. Luttges MW, Kelly PT, Gerren RA: Degenerative changes in mouse sciatic nerves: electrophoretic and electrophysiological characterization. *Exp Neurol* 50:706–733, 1976.

25. Triano JJ, Luttges MW: Nerve irritation: a possible model of sciatic neuritis. *Spine* 7:129–136, 1982.

26. Kleynhans AM: Vascular changes occurring in the cervical musculocutaneous system. *J Can Chiropractic Assoc,* 19–21, 1970.

27. Palmateer DC: Greater occipital-trigeminal syndrome. *J Clin Chiropractic* (arch ed), 46–48, Winter 1972.

28. Zeoli NJ: Anatomical and pathological consideration of the circle of Willis. *Dig Chiropractic Econ,* 44–45, November/December 1971.

29. Goldstein M (ed): *The Research Status of Spinal Manipulative Therapy.* Washington, DC, Government Printing Office, 1975.

30. Buerger AA, Tobis JS (eds): *Approaches to the Validation of Manipulation Therapy.* Springfield, IL, Charles C Thomas, 1977.

31. Korr I (ed): *Neurobiologic Mechanisms in Manipulative Therapy.* New York, Plenum, 1978.

32. Haldeman S (ed): *Modern Developments in the Principles and Practice of Chiropractic.* New York, Appleton-Century-Crofts, 1980.

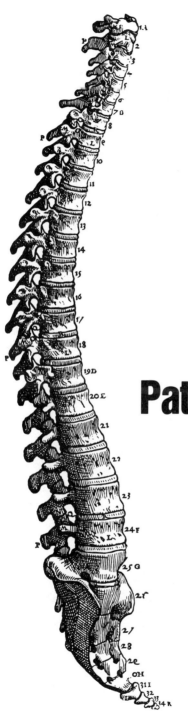

Section 2

Chiropractic Theories of Subluxation Pathophysiology

The microbe is nothing,
the soil is everything.

Louis Pasteur

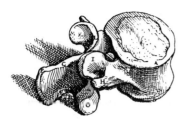

Chapter 5

Intervertebral Subluxation Hypothesis

Since its inception, the chiropractic profession has generally agreed with its founder, D. D. Palmer (1), that subluxations may be caused by acute trauma (e.g., strenuous posture) and poisons and other insults (2–5). That trauma in the form of accidents and even postural stresses may result in subluxations and/or arthroses of the spinal column has also been recognized by the medical profession (6–9). If the medical profession does not recognize that poisons may result in subluxations of vertebrae, it has certainly been documented that infections of various kinds may cause reflex spinal subluxations by some viscerosomatic pathway(s) (10–16).

Many other probable causes of subluxation have generally been underemphasized through the years in the chiropractic literature. These may help to explain why correction of the subluxation is not permanent in many cases (e.g., disc degeneration, unilateral arch defects, ligamentous damage, and erosive arthritides) (10–12, 17–19).

That intervertebral subluxations are a common occurrence is an idea accepted within the chiropractic profession; this idea in itself is a hypothesis that some within the medical profession would refute (20). Many nonpartisan medical authors, however, have reported the causes, development, and progress of intervertebral subluxations. A case can then be made that the medical profession itself has documented to some degree the *pathogenesis* of the various subluxations. In this text, the hypothesis that a wide variety of causes and types of subluxations are of relatively frequent occurrence in the general population is referred to as the *intervertebral subluxation* hypothesis. (It is acknowledged that there are subluxations that would not fall into the category of "intervertebral," but inclusion of these would be beyond the scope of our presentation.) This chapter focuses on the various reports and the various causes of subluxations in an effort to elucidate the intervertebral subluxation hypothesis. Before this review, however, a discussion of the principal methods that chiropractors use to differentiate subluxations will be helpful.

Spinography in Chiropractic

Spinography has been used extensively in the chiropractic profession; in fact its use was pioneered by B. J. Palmer (*spinography* is the term for radiographs taken while the patient is standing upright) (21). Spinographic examination of the spine is necessary in order to assess the postural and biomechanical integrity of the spine for indicators of intervertebral subluxations (22–24). Various analytical techniques may be used for visual identification of spinal subluxations on radiographs (Table 4.1) (22). It should be noted that according to our definition (see Chapter 3), determination of a spinal subluxation cannot be made from spinographic examination alone but can only be made by roentgenographic and neurologic criteria combined. It is the chiropractic viewpoint that postural status is a major factor in the pathogenesis of subluxations and that spinography is therefore the method of choice for its analysis (25–29).

Posture and Biped Man

One reason for the high incidence of spinal subluxations is associated with the evolutionary theory of development of man from a quadruped to a biped (30). The quadruped animal's skeleton is built like a cantilever bridge. The vertebrae form an arch which is supported by the four limbs; in this case the trunk and abdomen are the load that is supported and suspended by the well-balanced arch (31). According to the theory of evolution, man developed an upright stance or became biped. According to proponents of this theory, in order to accommodate to this new mechanical imbalance, man developed several anteroposterior (AP) curves. This proposed evolutionary scene is replayed during infancy, when the first or primary single-arch curve is broken into the secondary lordotic curves as the child learns to hold his head up and as the child begins to walk (32). Because of the biped

Table 5.1. Indicators and/or diagnostic roentgenographic findings in cases of intervertebral subluxation[a]

Analytic technique	Applicable region
Cervical subluxation evaluation	
Atlantodental interval	C1–C2
Incongruent triangles of atlas	C1–C2
Parallel lines of odontoid	C1–C2
Horizontal lines of atlas	C1
Horizontal lines of axis	C2
George's line	C1–C7
Periodontoid space	C1
Width of lateral mass	C1
Cervical hyperflexion-extension	C1–C7
Facet surface evaluation	C1–C7
Thoracic subluxation evaluation	
Body lamina junction system	T1–L5
Pedicle system	T1–L5
McNabb's line	T1–L5
Lumbar subluxation evaluation	
Hadley's "S" curve	L1–L5
George's line	L1–L5
Anterior body alignment	L1–L5
Intervertebral space narrowing	L1–L5
Hourglass indentation of IVF[b]	L1–L5
Approximation of spinous processes	L1–L5
Gapping and/or imbrication of facets	L1–L5
McNabb's line	L1–L5
Abnormal lumbar body angle	L1–L5

[a] From MacRae J: *Roentgenometrics in Chiropractic.* Toronto, published privately, 1974 (22).
[b] IVF, intervertebral foramen.

stance, man has developed the abililty to perform tasks that no other animal is capable of, but this freedom has been gained at a cost to his spine. For example, his lumbar vertebrae have been remodeled with a thicker edge anteriorly and a thinner edge posteriorly. Although this condition provides him with a greater range of motion, it also weakens the low back, which gives him a higher frequency of lumbar lesions (subluxation) (33).

Beyond the postural difficulty associated with this upright stance is the difficulty brought on when a person does not maintain this stance. Jackson (34) reported that occupations which require prolonged cervical hyperflexion or hyperextension or that require prolonged or repeated rotation or lateral bending of the neck may result in symptoms of foraminal encroachment. Perhaps more interesting is her finding that unilateral subluxations may occur when a person turns over in bed during sleep, with the neck muscles relaxed. Her findings indicate that although an upright posture has its inherent weaknesses, an improper posture presents even more difficulties. Certainly, according to these researchers (30–34), postural stresses are a major factor in the pathogenesis of subluxations.

Trauma

From the medical profession there is ample acknowledgment that trauma can cause subluxations. Hadley (10) recognized the occurrence of unilateral forward and rotary subluxations in the cervical spine when the patient's head is turned in an unguarded moment during an auto accident. Jacobson and Adler (7) reported that injuries to the atlas-axis joint may result in subluxations there. Their patients included those in auto accidents and one who fell down a staircase. Maigne (35), in a review of the literature, reported that the posterior branches of the spinal nerves are affected by any derangement of the posterior joints. He claimed that acute or chronic derangement may result in traction on the nerves; furthermore, other factors such as edema, periarticular hematoma, or ligamentocapsular tears may be involved. That dislocations at the atlas-axis level may be caused by trauma is also recognized by Wollin and Botterell (36). They cite cases in which injury was due to falls, blows to the head, auto accidents, and forced flexion and twisting of the neck during sporting events. Hughes (8) reported that blows to the head may result in cervical subluxation. He stated that hyperflexion of the cervical spine may tear the interspinous and dorsal column ligaments; the annulus fibrosus of intervertebral discs may also be torn. Sunderland (17) called attention to acute traumata affecting the spinal nerve roots when neighboring structures are displaced or deformed. Braakman and Penning (9) documented the case of a 12-year-old boy who developed an anterior C2-C3 subluxation on diving into shallow water. Kovacs (37) reported on cervical subluxations resulting from traumata or chondrosis. Seletz (6) reported that in whiplash injuries, a momentary posterior subluxation occurs and sometimes persists; he believed, however, that persistent symptoms are the result of nerve and blood vessel involvement. Seletz also believed that the axis is especially vulnerable in whiplash injuries. Other medicolegal authorities have now accepted that subluxations may occur in whiplash injuries; one has suggested that 90% of nerve root compression is due to whiplash injury and to subsequent subluxation and foraminal occlusion (38). In addition, cases of trauma resulting in lumbar and sacral subluxations have also been reported in the medical literature (10, 39, 40). Finally, Warwick and Williams (41) cited pregnancy as an event that may induce pelvic rotational subluxations, and Lounavaara (42) cited traumatic birth as a cause of subluxation in the newborn infant. Although chiropractors have generally believed that trauma is the most significant single cause of subluxations, medical researchers, however, have implicated many other factors.

Disc Degeneration

The intervertebral disc is a factor in the etiology of subluxations which cannot be overlooked. The disc is composed of a semigelatinous nucleus pulposus center (a network of collagen fibrils supporting a protein polysaccharide gel complex) and a surrounding dense annulus fibrosus (interlacing fibers of collagen attached to the adjacent vertebral bodies) (10, 41, 43). The discs are avascular (except for their periphery which may receive a supply from nearby blood vessels) and thus receive their nourishment from the adjacent vertebrae by diffusion (41). Normally, through the second decade of life, the discs are strong enough that traumata displace the vertebrae and not the discs (41). Yet, the natural aging process takes it toll on the structure; one of the first changes is deterioration of the nucleus pulposus and replacement of it with coarse collagen fibrils (10, 41, 43, 44). As this occurs, the disc loses some of its water content, which decreases the intradiscal pressure. This allows the cartilage plates to come closer together, with resultant discal bulging (10, 44). Normally, the nucleus pulposus acts as a hydrostatic ball bearing, supporting and cushioning the spine; these changes, however, promote instability and more thinning and bulging (10, 44). Instead of the nucleus pulposus carrying the superimposed weight, the annulus

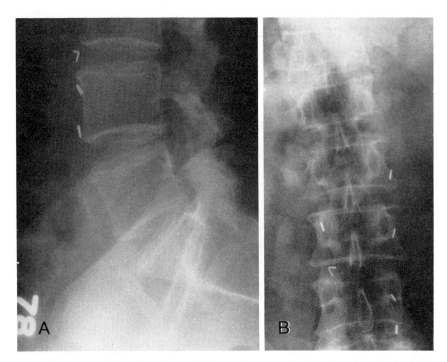

Figure 5.1. Radiographs of a middle-aged man who presented with objective signs of sciatica. The fifth lumbar vertebra is seen subluxating posteriorly on the sacrum, with a minor degree of L5-S1 disc narrowing *(A)*. Minor osteoarthritic changes include only minor lipping spurs and sclerosis of the lumbosacral apophyseal joints. The AP view *(B)* shows development of a simple scoliosis, the postural factor. The overall picture is that of developing lumbosacral instability, and future development of chronic L5 subluxation and/or spondylosis and chronic lumbar osteoarthritis (degenerative joint disease) is to be expected. (The metal clips seen in these radiographs are the result of vascular surgery).

fibrosus must increasingly perform this function. Tension is then placed on the longitudinal ligaments due to the discal bulging, and this may stimulate the production of bony spurs to stabilize the joint (10, 44). From the third decade of life on, injury, postural stresses, and trauma enhance this process (10, 41, 43–45). Therefore, it has been documented that disc degeneration, thinning, and bulging occur as a result of trauma and the general aging process. In addition, scoliosis will cause even more degenerative changes and spur formations to develop (10) (Figures 5.1 and 5.2).

The literature is replete with references to the effects of disc degeneration. Hadley (10) noted that if the disc becomes thinned

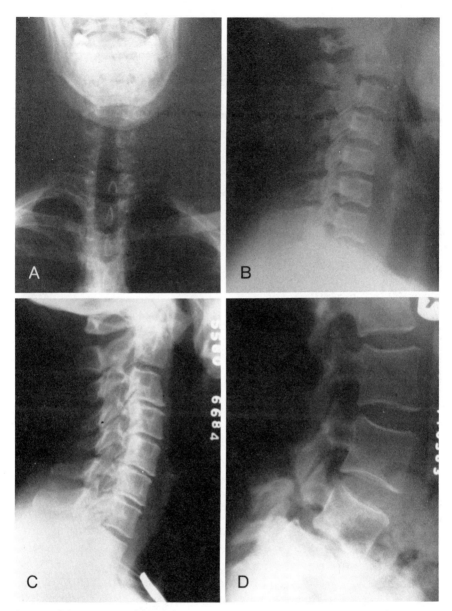

Figure 5.2, A–D. Radiographic examination can reveal subtle postural deviations *(A)* and traumatic injury such as whiplash with resultant so-called reversed
cervical curvature *(B)*. The young man who was left unconscious after he was
struck by a collapsing roof has developed significant degenerative joint disease
at the level of reversal subluxation (the C3-C4 vertebral motor unit) less than 3
years after the accident *(C)*. A defect in the pars interarticularis permits spondylolisthesis of the L5 vertebra in an x-ray *(D)* of a young woman who developed
severe radiculitis after she fell from a horse. The final result of trauma, postural
faults, chronic unreduced subluxation, etc., is often found to be severe multiple
spondylosis (degenerative joint disease) *(E)* as well as chronic postural imbalance *(F)* with clinical signs of permanent impairment.

41

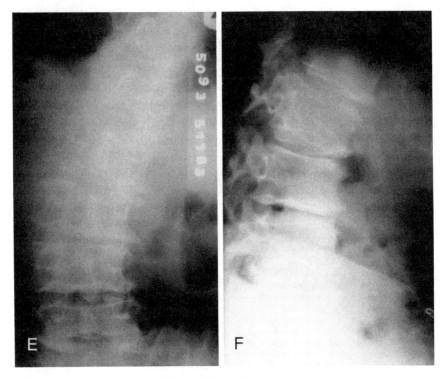

Figure 5.2, *E* and *F*.

in the lumbar region due to degeneration and, if the posterior articulations of the vertebrae remain intact, the superior vertebra will likely displace posteriorly (posterior subluxation or retrospondylolisthesis). Epstein et al. (39) reported on 15 patients who experienced sciatica. Disc herniation was not found in any of these patients, but nerve root entrapment in the lateral recess beneath the superior articular facet of the inferior vertebra was documented operatively. They concluded that the patients' symptoms were caused by trauma, which resulted in disc thinning that allowed posterior subluxations to occur. Sunderland (17) recognized disc thinning as a predisposing factor to subluxation in both the lower cervical and the lower lumbar spine:

> Narrowing of the intervertebral disc would lead to subluxation of the joint so that the superior articular process of the subjacent vertebra would move upwards toward the pedical of the vertebra above, thereby encroaching on that part of the foramen containing the nerve.

Smith (46) recognized diminishing thickness of the intervertebral disc as a secondary factor in the etiology of a posterior displacement. It can therefore be assumed from the literature that disc degeneration, especially when combined with trauma or postural stress, can result in posterior subluxation (displacement, retrolisthesis, retrospondylolisthesis) of the vertebral body above the discopathy when it occurs in the lower cervical or lower lumbar spines.

Erosive Arthritides

The erosive arthritides have also been implicated as causes of subluxation, especially in the cervical spine. The primary disease now clearly linked to upper cervical subluxation is *rheumatoid arthritis.* In *Dorland's Medical Dictionary* (50), this disease is defined as

> a chronic disease of the joints, usually polyarticular, marked by inflammatory changes in the synovial membranes and articular structures and by atrophy and rarefaction of the bones. In late stages[,] deformity and ankylosis develop. The cause is unknown, but autoimmune mechanisms and virus infection have been postulated.

It has been pointed out that atlas-axis subluxation and upward translocation of the odontoid are found in one fourth of all patients with rheumatoid arthritis (19). Rana et al. (19) found that 41 of 49 such patients had subluxations and 8 others had upward translocation of the odontoid. Davidson et al. (18) found atlas-axis subluxation in a case of brain stem compression. Others have noted that rheumatoid arthritis may cause atlas-axis or other cervical subluxations, and still others have implicated other erosive arthritides (including rheumatoid spondylitis and spondylitis deformans) as etiologies of subluxation (10, 47, 48). The mode of pathology is thought to be some unknown factor that causes a destructive synovitis of the atlas-axis articulations. This allows the atlas to subluxate, and in some cases the odontoid becomes translocated (48). Many of these authors reported that brain stem compression accompanies the subluxation or translocation of the odontoid with subsequent bulbar dysfunction; the findings of these authors is discussed in Chapter 7.

Infections

Various authors have recognized that infections commonly are complicated by subluxations (10–16). Grogono (11) reported on a patient suffering from forward subluxation of the atlas on the axis, which occurred 1 week after tonsillectomy. The 4-year-old boy also had a retropharyngeal abscess; he lay on his bed with the neck flexed and the head buried in a pillow, complaining of neck stiffness. Grogono reported on another patient (a 10-year-old girl) with anterior subluxation of the atlas which developed 1 week after an attack of sore throat. Sullivan (13) recognized the occurrence of subluxation mainly with inflammatory lesions of the neck, rheumatic fever, cervical gland infection, pharyngitis, retropharyngeal abscess, influenza, rheumatoid arthritis, and tonsillectomy. Grogono (11) claimed that spontaneous rotary dislocation (subluxation) was the most common type of lesion to affect the atlas and axis. Hess et al. (12) reported on atlas-axis dislocations in which trauma had not occurred recently but inflammatory foci were hypothesized as the initial cause. Hadley (10) also has recognized the role of inflammation in the pathogenesis of subluxation.

Recent reports (15, 16) of atlantoaxial subluxation following oral, head, and neck surgery have been detailed. Atlantoaxial subluxation, following pharyngoplasty, and subsequent infection, following otitis media without surgery and following surgical repair of choanal atresia and adenoidectomy, have been reported. Hypotheses as to the mechanism of displacement because of inflammation are not clearly presented by these authors. Ligaments, muscles, and associated structures of the vertebral motor unit, however, may be significant in if not critical to the pathogenesis in these cases.

Congenital and Developmental Factors

Various congenital and developmental structural faults have been associated with subluxation. It is generally recognized that a defect in the isthmus of the neural arch in the lumbar region, or separation of the pars interarticularis, may be complicated by a type of subluxation known as spondylolisthesis (anterior subluxation, anterolisthesis). It was formerly thought that this break was due to some congenital deformity, but in more recent studies Hadley (10) has pointed out that not a single case of congenital defect in the isthmus has been found among some 600 fetal, stillborn, and newborn subjects. Hadley has concluded that the problem is developmental and results from a combination of pressure (as the normal lumbar lordosis develops) and trauma. Ligaments and muscles have also been mentioned as factors important in the pathogenesis of subluxation. Damage to the posterior interspinous ligament, according to cadaver studies by Hadley (10), may allow a forward or anterior subluxation to occur. Moreover, complex computer programming of spinal ligaments and spinal and paraspinal muscles may reveal specific soft-tissue weaknesses that result in subluxations (49). Other structural problems may give rise to subluxation that are congenital in nature. Smith (46) reported that in many people the lumbar articulating facets face more anteroposteriorly than laterally, which predisposes that vertebra to posterior displacement. Thus, there are congenital and developmental factors that should be considered when the pathogenesis of subluxations is differentiated.

Discussion

As can be seen, there are indeed a wide variety of acknowledged causes and types of intervertebral subluxations that have been cited in the medical literature. It has been shown that subluxations may occur from postural, nontraumatic, traumatic, degenerative, infectious, developmental, and congenital faults. It has also been proposed that, as humans, we are susceptible structurally to low back subluxation by our very evolution.

It must be kept in mind that there is an interplay between the causative factors cited in this chapter and that a combination of more than one factor may be precipitating the intervertebral subluxation. Turek (44) points out that excessive imposed weight, an acute lumbosacral angle, degenerative changes associated with advancing age, loss of the intervertebral disc, chronic occupational postural strains, and a vertical disposition of the articular facets are predisposing factors that may encourage tearing of the capsular ligaments and lumbar subluxation.

The wide variety of causative factors—from subluxations following traumatic birth to subluxations due to twisting during sleep—

and the fact that the general population deals with one or more of these stresses daily suggest that the intervertebral subluxation hypothesis is valid as it has been broadly presented.

Summary

The intervertebral subluxation hypothesis is probably correct in that a wide variety of causative or predisposing factors may promote the onset of the lesion with some frequency in the general population. That postural, nontraumatic, and traumatic factors cause intervertebral subluxations makes the entire population susceptible to the lesion (6–10, 17, 35–42). Disc degeneration predisposes especially the elderly (10, 41, 43–45). Infections have been shown to induce the lesion in children, and erosive arthritides may cause subluxations in yet another group of individuals (10–14, 18, 47, 48). Congenital and developmental causes have also been implicated (10, 34, 46).

References

1. Palmer DD: *The Science, Art and Philosphy of Chiropractic.* Portland, OR, Portland Printing House, 1910.
2. Palmer BJ: *The Science of Chiropractic.* Davenport, IA, Palmer School of Chiropractic, 1908.
3. Dintenfass J: *Chiropractic: A Modern Way to Health.* New York, Pyramid, 1970.
4. Verner JR: *The Science and Logic of Chiropractic.* Brooklyn, Cerasoli, 1941.
5. Pharoah DO: *Chiropractic Orthopody.* Davenport, IA, Palmer School of Chiropractic, 1956.
6. Seletz E: Whiplash injuries. *JAMA* 168:1750–1755. 1958.
7. Jacobson G, Adler DC: Examination of the atlantoaxial joint following injury with particular emphasis on rotational subluxation. *Am J Roentgenol* 76:1081–1094, 1956.
8. Hughes JT: Spinal cord trauma. In: *Greenfield's Neuropathology.* London, Edward Arnold, 1976, pp 665–666.
9. Braakman R, Penning L: Injuries to the cervical spine. In Vinken PJ, Bruyn GW (eds): *Handbook of Clinical Neurology.* Injuries to the spinal cord part 1. New York, Elsevier, 1976, vol 25, pp 341–345.
10. Hadley LA: *Anatomico Roentgenographic Studies of the Spine.* Springfield, IL, Charles C Thomas, 1964.
11. Grogono BJS: Injuries of the atlas and axis. *Br J Bone Joint Surg* 36B:397–410, 1954.
12. Hess JH, Bronstein IP, Abelson SM: Atlanto-axial dislocations unassociated with trauma and secondary to inflammatory foci in the neck. *Am J Dis Child* 49:137, 1935.
13. Sullivan AW: Subluxation of the atlanto-axial joint. *J Pediatr* 35:451–464, 1949.
14. Hansen TA, et al: Subluxation of the cervical vertebra due to pharyngitis. *South Med J* 66:427–430, 1973.
15. Hopla DM, Mazur JM, Bass RM: Cervical vertebrae subluxation. *Laryngoscope* 93:1155–1159, 1983.
16. Robinson PH, DeBoer A: La maladie de Grisel: a rare occurrence of "spontaneous" atlanto-axial subluxation after pharyngoplasty. *Br J Plast Surg* 34:319–321, 1981.
17. Sunderland S: Anatomical perivertebral influences on the intervertebral foramen. In

Goldstein M (ed): *The Research Status of Spinal Manipulative Therapy.* Washington, DC, Government Printing Office, 1975, pp 129–140.

18. Davidson RC, Horn JR, Herndon JH, Grin OD: Brain stem compression in rheumatoid arthritis. *JAMA* 238:2633–2634, 1977.

19. Rana NA, Hancock DO, Taylor AR, Hill AGS: Atlanto-axial subluxation and upward translocation of the odontoid process in rheumatoid arthritis. *Am J Bone Joint Surg* 55A:1304, 1973.

20. Shapiro R: Discussion: comments on subluxation—pathophysiology and diagnosis. In Goldstein M (ed): *The Research Status of Spinal Manipulative Therapy.* Washington, DC, Government Printing Office, 1975, pp 265–266.

21. Gibbons RW: The evolution of chiropractic: medical and social protest in America. In Haldeman S (ed): *Modern Developments in the Principles and Practice of Chiropractic.* New York, Appleton-Century-Crofts, 1980, pp 3–24.

22. MacRae J: *Roentgenometrics in Chiropractic.* Toronto, published privately, 1974.

23. Howe JW: The role of x-ray findings in structural diagnosis. In Goldstein M (ed): *The Research Status of Spinal Manipulative Therapy.* Washington, DC, Government Printing Office, 1975, pp 239–247.

24. Phillips RB: The use of x-rays in spinal manipulative therapy. In Haldeman S (ed): *Modern Developments in the Principles and Practice of Chiropractic.* New York, Appleton-Century-Crofts, 1980, pp 3–24.

25. Homewood AE: *The Neurodynamics of the Vertebral Subluxation.* Thornhill, Ontario, published privately, 1973.

26. Drum DC: The vertebral motor unit and intervertebral foramen. In Goldstein M (ed): *The Research Status of Spinal Manipulative Therapy.* Washington, DC, Government Printing Office, 1975, pp 63–75.

27. Pettibon BR: Biomechanical research of the spine. *Today's Chiropractic* 5:34–35, 1976.

28. Watkins RJ, Shrubb E: Vasodilation neurology. *Today's Chiropractic* 7:24,44, 1978.

29. Shepherd WP: Differentiating spinal subluxations from strain distortions or compensations. *Dig Chiropractic Econ* 18:64–67, 1975.

30. Wright HM: *Perspectives in Osteopathic Medicine.* Kirksville, MO, Kirksville College of Osteopathic Medicine, 1976.

31. Gregory WK: The bridge that walks. *Natural Hist* 39:33–48, 1937.

32. Moore KL: *Before We Are Born.* Philadelphia, Saunders, 1974.

33. Krogman WM: The scars of human evolution. *Sci Am* 185:54–57, 1951.

34. Jackson R: *The Cervical Syndrome.* Springfield, IL, Charles C Thomas, 1978.

35. Maigne R: *Orthopedic Medicine, A New Approach to Vertebral Manipulations.* Springfield, IL, Charles C Thomas, 1972.

36. Wollin DG, Botterell EH: Symmetrical forward luxation of the atlas. *Am J Roentgenol* 79:575–583, 1958.

37. Kovacs A: Subluxation and deformation of the cervical apophyseal joints. *Acta Radiol* 43:1–15, 1955.

38. Berstein B: *Whiplash Its Medical-Legal Aspects.* Legal Medicine Institute, 1958.

39. Epstein JA, Epstein BS, Lavine LS, Carras R, Rosenthal AD, Sumner P: Sciatica caused by nerve root entrapment in the lateral recess: the superior facet syndrome. *J Neurosurg* 36:584–589, 1972.

40. Mennell J: *Back Pain.* Boston, Little, Brown & Co, 1960.

41. Warwick R, Williams PL (eds): *Gray's Anatomy,* ed 35(Br). Philadelphia, Saunders, 1973, pp 412–413.

42. Lounavaara KI: Forward subluxation of atlas following birth trauma. *Acta Pediatr* 37:341, 1949.

43. Boyd W: *A Textbook of Pathology,* ed 8. Philadelphia, Lea & Febiger, 1970, pp 1377–1379.

44. Turek SL: *Orthopedics: Principles and Their Application.* Philadelphia, Lippincott, 1967.
45. Meschan I: *Synopsis of Analysis of Roentgen Signs in General Radiology.* Philadelphia, Saunders, 1976.
46. Smith A: Posterior displacement of 5th L vertebra. *J Bone Joint Surg* 16:877–888, 1934.
47. Mathews JA: Atlanto-axial subluxation in rheumatoid arthritis: a five-year follow-up study. *Ann Rheum Dis* 33:526–531, 1974.
48. Latchaw RE, Meyer GW: Reiter disease with atlantoaxial subluxation. *Radiology* 126:303–304, 1978.
49. Suh CH: Biomechanical aspects of subluxation. In Goldstein M (ed): *The Research Status of Spinal Manipulative Therapy.* Washington, DC, Government Printing Office, 1975, pp 103–119.
50. Friel JP (ed): *Dorland's Illustrated Medical Dictionary,* ed 25. Philadelphia, Saunders, 1974, p 147.

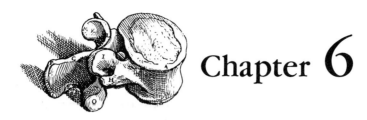

Chapter 6

Nerve Compression Hypothesis

*P*erhaps the most commonly recognized of the chiropractic theories is the one proposed by D. D. Palmer (1) who stated that a vertebra that was out of place could press on a spinal nerve and thereby increase or decrease its flow of nerve energy. Numerous other chiropractic authors have since commented on this idea, and it has become a source of dispute both within and outside the chiropractic profession (2–8). Although according to the original Palmer thesis this increased or decreased nerve energy constituted altered body tonus and therefore disease, we discuss the latter portion of his hypothesis as a component of the neurodystrophic hypothesis in Chapter 12. For the purpose of discussion, the *nerve compression* hypothesis is defined as the chiropractic hypothesis that intervertebral subluxations can interfere with the normal transmission of nerve energy (i.e., action potentials and other associated neural phenomena) by irritating or compressing the spinal nerve roots.

Hadley (9, 10) along with others (11–18) has documented that intervertebral subluxations are a cause of spinal nerve root compression. Moreover, to our knowledge Hadley is the only investigator to link the subluxation to specific nerve root pathology discovered during postmortem examination. Others (19–22) have linked disc herniation to nerve root pathology, and still other researchers (23, 24) have been working on an animal model for the subluxation, to study its effects *in vivo*. Luttges and his colleagues (25–28) at the University of Colorado have recently presented studies of the local pathophysiology of nerve root compression and damage following various types of injury to animal nerves (see also Chapter 10).

Duncan's (29) work in 1948 represented a landmark in nerve studies. Since then, other experimenters have shown in detail the pathophysiology of various types of nerve injury (28, 30–35). Attention has been directed to the susceptibility of nerve roots to compression by Gelfan and Tarlov (36) and Sharpless (37). These studies and the work of Sunderland (17, 38–40) and others (9, 10, 41–44) tend to refute the suggestion by Crelin (8) that spinal nerve roots cannot be compressed in patients with subluxation. In light of these and other findings, the all-or-none law along with a review of the contributions of these aforementioned scientists and medical doctors is considered in this chapter. Finally, from the literature a pathophysiological and clinical picture is presented which includes demyelination, degeneration, muscle atrophy, flaccid weakness, diminished or absent superficial and deep tendon reflexes, and a decrease of the compound action potential (9, 10, 19–22, 27–37, 45–47).

Compression or Irritation?

As Triano and Luttges (48) pointed out in discussion at the Ninth Annual Biomechanics Conference on the Spine, the typical chiropractic patient shows signs of paresthesia or pain, which can be traced to cervical or lumbar spinal derangements. These patients are actually reporting increased neural activity. Conversely, spinal nerve root compression would be expected to result in effects quite the opposite of those seen in the practitioner's office (i.e., spinal nerve root compression would be expected to decrease the function of the nerve fibers, which would result in decrements in the compound action potential as well as numbness or paralysis). Yet since the days of D. D. Palmer, some chiropractors have promulgated the nerve compression hypothesis to explain all of the many and varied effects of subluxations (2–6).

Palmer (1) himself was probably the first to suggest that there would be a clinically noticeable difference between mere "irritation" and "compression" of the spinal nerve roots. He stated that irritation of the nerves could result in hyperfunction and painful states. He said too that intervertebral subluxations could squeeze, compress, or pinch the outgoing nerves within the intervertebral foramen. Hence, Palmer developed his hypothesis that disease resulted from either too much or not enough nerve energy.

Several important questions are raised by his assertion: Can intervertebral subluxations alter the shape of intervertebral foramina? Is it possible for spinal nerves to become irritated or compressed because of this change? What might the clinical effects of this *subluxation pathophysiology* include? In order to answer these questions we will first examine Crelin's study of the intervertebral foramen as well as studies of the spinal nerve roots.

Crelin's "Test of Chiropractic Theory"

Nature has developed an amazing protective mechanism to safeguard against nerve compression even when subluxations cause foraminal encroachment. Of course, the first and second cervical nerve roots pass over the posterior arch of atlas and behind the medial margin of the axial articulating facets, respectively (17). The rest of the spinal nerve roots, however, must pass through the intervertebral foramina located bilaterally at each intersegmental level. The posterior nerve roots are thicker than the anterior roots, especially in the cervical area where the posterior nerve roots are three times as large. The nerve roots and their sheaths occupy between 35% and 50% of the total cross-sectional area of the intervertebral foramen, with the former figure pertaining especially to the dorsal foramina (40, 49). The remaining 50% to 65% of the foramen contains loose areolar connective and adipose tissue with the spinal artery, numerous veins, lymphatics, and the recurrent meningeal nerve (49). These latter contents provide the nerve roots with an ample cushion from the periosteal boundaries of the foramen.

This basic fact became the focus of attention when Crelin (8) studied the effects of gross rotational, compressive, and torsional forces on six fresh cadaver spines. Crelin, a well-recognized anatomist, entitled the study, "The First Scientific Test of Chiropractic Theory." He used a Mura volt-ohm-microampere meter on the first vertebral column (from a 35-year-old man) (8):

> The meter was used to determine whether the border of the intervertebral foramen came into contact with the spinal nerve when compressive, bending, or twisting forces were applied to the vertebral column. The wire from the positive pole of the meter was wrapped around the spinal nerve that was placed against one side of the intervertebral foramen; the wire from the negative pole of the meter

was placed against the opposite side of the foramen. The meter was set at 1,000 ohms, and if the wires barely touched each other[,] the recording needle would make a full swing across the face of the dial.

While the first spine was being tested, it became obvious that the nerve roots would never actually touch the bony foramen, according to Crelin; so the meter was disconnected. After testing the other spines, Crelin decided that the *nerve compression* hypothesis (which he called "chiropractic theory"—it should be noted, of course, that this is only one chiropractic theory) was false (8):

> This experimental study demonstrates conclusively that the subluxation of a vertebra as defined by chiropractic—the exertion of pressure on a spinal nerve which by interfering with the planned expression of Innate Intelligence produces pathology—does not occur.

Crelin may have thought that his experiment duplicated the true conditions under which nerve root compression or irritation might occur. Several phenomena in real life, however, make the spinal nerve roots susceptible to such damage; an analysis of the spinal nerve roots is therefore in order.

Spinal Nerve Roots

Nerve complex has been defined as the nerve roots, posterior root ganglion, and the spinal nerve together with their connective tissue coverings (17). Each pair of anterior and posterior nerve roots invaginate the dura and arachnoid mater to pass through the intervertebral foramina. The dura mater becomes the strong perineurial sheath for the spinal nerve that is formed by the fusion of the two roots just past the dorsal nerve root ganglia. The perineurium is continuous with the epineurium of the spinal nerve, and this combination increases the cross-sectional area of the spinal nerve, as opposed to the total cross-sectional area of the combined nerve roots. One important point then is that the nerve roots do not have the strong connective tissue sheaths (epineurial and perineurial) that support peripheral nerves (40).

Other factors indicate that the spinal nerve roots are more susceptible to irritation or compression than are the spinal nerves. For example, in humans the nerve roots are placed in tension by traction on peripheral nerves (49). Thus head and neck movements place tension on cervical nerve roots (17):

> With ventroflexion the nerve roots are tensed and the complex is drawn inwards and upwards toward the upper margin of the foramen;

in dorsal extension the complex is relaxed and returns to its original position. The nerve roots maximally involved in this way are the eighth cervical to the fifth thoracic, but ventroflexion of the cervical spine also tenses the lumbar and sacral nerve roots.

The elastic properties of the nerve roots allow them to accommodate such tension. Nerve roots do not display the tensile strength of their peripheral counterparts, however; studies have shown nerve roots to fail before peripheral nerves when nerve roots are tested under increasing tension (17, 39). Sunderland believes that this is due to structural differences; the nerve root fibers are arranged in parallel bundles with fewer enveloping collagen fibers than are found in peripheral nerve trunks. This is in addition to the previously mentioned fact that the nerve roots lack the connective tissue sheaths that support peripheral nerves.

The nerve roots of C4 to C7 are bound to the transverse processes of their respective vertebrae for protection against traction injury (17). For this reason, traction injuries that do not avulse the roots usually occur in the upper cervical spine, whereas traction injuries involving avulsion of nerve roots occur in the lower cervical spine where the nerve root is sheared from the transverse process (17). Hence, lower cervical traction injuries carry the added danger of spinal nerve root avulsion.

In examining the various postmortem and clinical studied concerning evidence of nerve root damage, Hadley (9) came to this conclusion:

> Any abnormal constriction in the size of a normal intervertebral foramen if not actually causing nerve root pressure, nervertheless decreases the reserve safety cushion space surrounding that nerve and may predispose to pressure. The subsequent development of radiculitis, edema, hemorrhage, additional disc pressure or movement of adjacent structures may be sufficient to produce radicular symptoms.

The significance of these postmortem findings are discussed later in this chapter. It is noteworthy, however, that Hadley (9, 10) found evidence that cervical and lumbar subluxations could produce foraminal encroachment that would cause or at least predispose the spinal nerve roots to compression (Figure 6.1). He also found that intervertebral subluxations could cause foraminal encroachment in the thoracic spine, but he determined that nerve root compression would be unlikely there due to the smaller diameters of the nerve roots (9, 10, 42, 43).

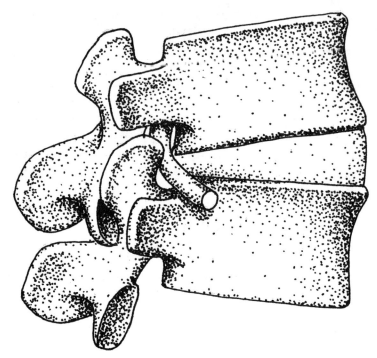

Figure 6.1. Schema illustrating susceptibility of the midlumbar nerve root to distortion (compression, stretch, deformation) after posterior subluxation of the articulating facets. Hadley (9, 10, 42, 43) was the first to demonstrate this phenomenon by postmortem research on human spines.

Other researchers have recognized the significance of foraminal encroachment in producing signs of nerve irritation or compression. Breig and Marions (41) studied 103 patients suspected of lumbosacral disc herniations and decided that nerve root compression would be likely at this site due to the anatomical and mechanical conditions. Rosomoff and Rossman (44) estimate that 75% of persons over 50 have some degree of narrowing of the cervical intervertebral foramina.

It has been proposed that some types of subluxations may result in venous congestion, which might affect neural elements and the sympathetic plexus. This chiropractic hypothesis remains largely unexplored, however (50–53).

In summary, there is a substantial amount of evidence to suggest that nerve roots are more mechanically predisposed to irritation or compression than are peripheral nerves. It has been reported that nerve roots lack the tensile strength of peripheral nerves and that they fail when deformed under increasing tension before their peripheral trunks (17, 39). It has also been reported that intervertebral subluxations may cause or at least predispose the nerve roots to irritation or compression in both cervical and lumbar levels (9, 10, 41–44). These weaknesses predispose the nerve roots to the very type of irritation or compression that might occur when subluxation results in foraminal encroachment.

These data contrast with the findings of Crelin (8), whose studies on cadaver spines—with their lifeless mechanics—provide little actual comparison to their living counterparts. Moreover, the fact that the data throughout this chapter deal with the localized pathophysiology of the intervertebral subluxation, as determined by postmortem, operative, and experimental evidence, suggests that Crelin's conclusions were highly inaccurate and misleading.

Postmortem Histological Examination

Postmortem examination of the spinal nerve roots following compression has been performed by some researchers. Hadley (9, 10) studied the pathophysiology of nerve root compression due to various causes including subluxation. Lindblom and Rexed (30) dissected 17 cadaver spines to examine the nerve roots in cases of dorsolateral disc herniation. These studies are very significant because they directly link subluxation and disc lesions, respectively, to nerve root damage and pathology.

Hadley found that disc herniations, exostoses, or subluxations may produce pressure on the dorsal nerve root. He found in some cases a marked fibrosis and thickening of the epineurium that attached the root to the foramen walls. Such nerves were removed only by sharp dissection (normally nerves may be removed by blunt dissection). Changes noted histologically included stages of both nerve degeneration and regeneration (9):

> Certain nerve bundles and ganglion cells were found flattened. Many Schwann tubules outlined by the neurilemma were empty of myelin and axones where the macrophages had removed these degenerated elements. In other sections of the same nerve bundle, these tubules were seen already filled with multiple rods of Schwann protoplasm and nuclei. . . . Some evidence of edema of the endoneurium was observed. Hemorrhage beneath the perineurium was found involving numerous roots in one specimen having adhesions about

those structures. Sclerosis of arterioles within the nerve bundle was also observed.

Hadley believed that the disc lesion was blamed too often as the cause of the nerve root pressure. He documented evidence of subluxations in the cervical, thoracic, and lumbar areas but believed that only subluxation in the cervical and lumbar areas could cause nerve encroachment (9, 10, 42, 43). He preferred to use conservative care first and surgery only when the former had received a thorough trial run.

Lindblom (19) found 60 nerve root compressions in 160 cadavers; these specimens were from patients aged 14 to 87 years. Most of the compressions (in the lumbar spine) were caused by dorsolateral protrusions against the lateral border of the intervertebral canal. In a follow-up study by Lindblom and Rexed (30), it was determined that compression of a spinal nerve root results in serious injury. Their findings, both macroscopically and microscopically, were generally in accord with those of Hadley. Lindblom and Rexed found cases in which the nerve roots were flattened or hollowed and cases in which the nerve and ganglion adhered to the protruding disc mass by dense connective tissue (separation was necessary with a knife). Of the 17 cadavers chosen for follow-up study, 44 segments were examined histologically by serial sectioning of the damaged nerves and of the corresponding normal nerves (30):

> The damage is most obvious in the ventral root bundles. . . . The basic effect of the compression is degeneration of a greater or lesser number of the nerve fibers. The damage does not occur as a massive, single trauma to the nerves but as many, repeated small traumata. Furthermore, each trauma is not restricted to a sharply localized point but exerts its effect over a relatively large area. As a result the degenerating nerve fibers are usually diffusely strewn all over the cross section in smaller or greater numbers in proportion to the severity and duration of the compression. Also[,] the standing of the degeneration varies from fiber to fiber, [with] some showing signs of a fresh [lesion], others of an earlier lesion.

Lindblom and Rexed were also in accord with Hadley on the clinical picture, with the characteristic feature being mixed degeneration and regeneration, depending on which fibers were most recently damaged. Degenerative fibers, when they were few, appeared as small patches with Schwann cell proliferation; large and small regenerated fibers were also present. With more degeneration, the damaged fibers formed a large "field" that surrounded isolated undamaged fibers. Lindblom and Rexed reported that damage to motor (ventral) roots was more severe than damage to sensory (dorsal) roots. In addition, damage to the spinal ganglion was even more prominent in cases of compression (30):

> Instead of showing the normal round cross section[,] it may sometimes appear as a crescent or sickle. This general deformation also influences the cells themselves, which become flattened and deformed, especially near the compressed margin of the ganglion. Some of these cells show definite signs of atrophy and changed staining reactions.

In nearly every case there was a direct relationship between the degree of compression and the extent of damage to the nerve root.

Thus, the only postmortem studies (human) available indicate that subluxation is a factor in the compression of nerve roots and that the subsequent pathology depends on the severity of compression. Pathophysiological features at the site of subluxation might include demyelination and degeneration of an individual fiber or groups of fibers, edema of the endoneurium, sclerosis of arterioles within the nerve bundle, and damage to the spinal ganglion itself (9, 10, 30, 42, 43).

Operative Confirmation

Various investigators have documented during surgery that nerve root compression may result in a variety of symptoms and clinical findings as well as damage to the nerve. In a classic study by Eaton (45), the diagnoses in 100 consecutive cases of nerve root pain were compared. Several important clinical aspects were documented. First, there was a characteristic distribution of the pain (segmental or dermatomal). Second, pain was intensified by increasing the intra-abdominal and intrathoracic pressure (by coughing, sneezing, lifting, defecation, etc.). Third, stretching of the nerve roots (by bending the neck, stooping, straight leg raising, and the Lasègue test) produced or intensified the pain. These clinical findings were based on the study that involved nerve compression lesions and diseases of known and unknown origin. Epstein et al. (46, 47) have shown that with L5 or S1 spinal nerve root compression, symptoms of pain, intermittent claudi-cation (pain, tension, and weakness in limbs during walking) with increasing weakness or numbness, leg weakness, and sensory changes may be presented. Furthermore, clinical findings might include sciatica, limitation of back mobility, paravertebral muscle spasm, scoliosis, depressed or absent ankle reflexes, diminished or absent patellar reflexes, weakness and atrophy of certain mus-cles (especially those affecting extensor hallucis longus and an-terior tibial muscle groups), and paresis of the quadriceps and hamstrings (46, 47). According to Epstein et al., a positive Lasègue sign will be indicative of sciatica, and electromyography seems to be an accurate clinical tool for determination of nerve root entrap-ment. Frykholm (54) further documents findings of pain, numb-ness, paresthesias, and muscle weakness resulting from nerve root compression. Breig and Marions (41) believe that disc herniation produces tension rather than compression on the nerves, but they recognize the subsequent damage that occurs. In their studies of 103 cases of suspected lumbosacral disc herniations, they rea-soned that the neurological signs encountered were due to such tension or stretching of the nerve roots. Thus, the operative data suggest that a wide variety of subjective and clinical findings may result from nerve compression and hence subluxation (41, 45–47, 54). Yet, postmortem and operative findings are only part of the pathophysiological picture.

Experimental Studies

A number of researchers have experimentally studied the effects of nerve trunk and root compression in animals. Denny-Brown and Brenner (31) reviewed the literature and found references to paralysis resulting from even minimal mechanical trauma. They endeavored to establish this histologically. They also wanted to determine the relationship between pressure on nerves and the onset and duration of subsequent paralysis. Two sets of experi-ments were carried out. In one set of experiments, it took direct pressure ranging from 160 to 1200 mm Hg and applied for several to 90 minutes to block the conduction of cat sciatic nerve trunks. These experiments revealed great variations in latency from case to case (i.e., the delay in failure of conduction). Thus, the expla-nation was presented that at lower pressures the nerves continued to conduct impulses because adjacent vessels supplied the needed oxygen. Denny-Brown and Brenner concluded that when higher pressures were applied to the nerve, conduction block occurred as these adjacent vessels and tissues became ischemic. Yet, no damage to the nerves was evident histologically, even in nerves that had not returned to normal conduction after 2 hours. In another set of experiments, the authors applied an infant's blood pressure cuff (folded to give a width of only 6 cm) to the thigh contralateral to the already-operated-on thigh. This "tourniquet paralysis" resulted in definite histological changes, including early vacuolation and swelling of axis-cylinders and vacuolation of myelin. After 48 hours, myelin began disappearing at the nodes of Ranvier. The axis-cylinders no longer retained the argentophil property (a property of having affinity for silver and chromium salts). Interestingly, repair continued long after normal nerve conduction had returned.

Duncan's (29) findings were in accord with those of Denny-Brown and Brenner. Yet, his research resulted in a more detailed picture of nerve compression pathophysiology. Duncan's objective was to mimic—by utilizing the right sciatic nerve trunks of eight rats—the condition that is encountered with chronic nerve root compression in the intervertebral foramen. Ligatures were fitted loosely around the sciatic nerves of young rats (.40 cotton thread in four rats and .36 tantalum wire in the others). Additional experiments in which tantalum sleeves were utilized with four kittens and with young rats proved largely unsuccessful. Six to 7 months later, the rats were sacrificed due to the development of motor weakness in the affected limbs. Histologically, it was found that there was a tremendous adaptability of the nerves to gradual compression. It was noted that this probably accounts for the discrepancies sometimes encountered at the intervertebral foramen (where one nerve root is distorted with little actual destruction, and another is barely distorted but markedly destroyed). Edema was present both proximal and distal to the ligation. This, too, was in accord with previous observations. Complete demyelination occurred at the zone of ligation, along with slight reduction in the axis-cylinder diameter. Distal to the ligation, up to 25% of the fibers became demyelinated without muscle impairment. Growth distal to the application of the ligature was retarded up to 50%. There was, in addition, reduction in the axis-cylinder diameter and thinning of the myelin sheaths both immediately proximal and distal to the ligature. Thus, the findings he presented further detailed the pathophysiology of nerve compression.

One study of importance to the chiropractic profession was that of Dyck (32). For a century, researchers studied the phenomenon of so-called hypertrophic interstitial neuropathy without understanding the cause. Dyck made repeated applications of a pressure cuff apparatus to rat sciatic nerve trunks for 1 to 2½ hours each time. The intervals between application ranged from 11 to 63 days. A pressure of between 120 and 130 mm Hg was applied. In this way, demyelination and remyelination occurred repeatedly in the same axons. This is similar to the condition Hadley (9, 10) found in nerves following compression and associated with subluxation. Lindblom and Rexed (30) also noted degeneration of some fibers with regeneration of others in the same nerve following compression by disc herniation. Experimentally, Dyck produced the "onion-bulb" formations characteristic of hypertrophic neuropathy by forcing this continual demyelination and remyelination. The onion-bulb formation consists of myelinated fibers in the center, with an inner lamellae composed of circumferentially oriented Schwann cells separated by longitudinally oriented collagen fibrils and with an outer lamellae made up of fibroblasts. Dyck thus holds the view that the onion-bulbs of hypertrophic neuropathy are a response to repeated segmental demyelination and remyelination. From the studies already presented, it should by evident that subluxation plays a role in nerve compression and hence the degenerative and regenerative processes that would give rise to onion-bulb formation. A direct relationship between subluxation and hypertrophic neuropathy, however, has yet to be documented.

Using a modification of the Duncan (29) technique (which was largely unsuccessful), Aguayo et al. (33) applied siliconized rubber tubes to the medial popliteal branch of the sciatic nerve of young rabbits, which restricted the growth of the nerves. Gradual constriction of the nerves eventually resulted in slowing of motor conduction across the constricted portion and in segmental demyelination in and around the area of compression. Histologic and electrophysiologic analysis revealed, however, that in the 17 animals included in the long-term studies, there were no indications of limb weakness, change in tonus, or atrophy of muscle.

Leg lengths preconstriction and postconstriction were compared. No appreciable difference between the control leg and the constricted leg was noted, and thus the findings of Duncan (29) (retardation of growth in the leg with a restricted nerve) were questioned. Furthermore, there was no appreciable difference in the internodal distance between control and constricted nerves (nodes of Ranvier) except at the site of constriction. The characteristic demyelination and remyelination picture was noted, which is in accord with the findings of Hadley (9, 10), Lindblom and Rexed (30), and Dyck (32). Aguayo et al. (33) concluded that chronic compression changes are not simply the result of nerve thinning and displacement of substance in the area of constriction. Instead, Aguayo et al. believed, the main factor in compression pathophysiology was the demyelination.

In an experiment similar to that of Denny-Brown and Brenner (31), Fowler et al. (34) blocked the conduction of sciatic nerve in baboons by application of an infant's sphygmomanometer cuff around the knee. Cuff pressures of 1,000 or 500 mm Hg were maintained for 1 to 3 hours in the various animals. Although the majority of findings were in accord with Denny-Brown and Brenner (31), several interesting findings were noted. Even after release of the cuff (within 24 hours), there was a reduction in conduction velocity of the nerve. This reduction occurred before the onset of demyelination and must be explained by other factors, such as occlusion of the nodes of Ranvier and the paranodal invaginations present for several days after compression. Perhaps even more importantly, the conduction velocity decreased through the compressed segment but became normal again after the zone of compression was passed. This was true both during and after compression with use of a pneumatic cuff, according to the experiments of both Denny-Brown and Brenner (31) and Fowler et al. (34).

Further experimentation on the effects of compression on nerve conduction velocity was completed recently by Rainer et al. (35). The ulnar nerves of 12 dogs were studied. Compression of the experimental nerves was obtained by the application of 500- and 900-gm weights. The duration of nerve compression rarely exceeded 2 minutes—long enough for the recording of stimulus and response. A significant drop in conduction velocities was recorded. Rainer et al. conjectured that the findings could be secondary to the effect of compression on various types of fibers within the trunk or could be due to transient ischemia secondary to compression, along with disturbed electrolyte balance.

Opponents of chiropractic theory have pointed to these studies by neurophysiologists to document their position (7). The studies show that nerve conduction slows in a zone of compression but returns to normal after the zone (31, 34, 35). It must be remembered, however, that these studies are of peripheral nerve trunks, not of the roots which have inherent weaknesses (38–40). Furthermore, modern studies of nerve root conduction suggest an entirely different picture (36, 37, 55).

Probably the first important study by neurophysiologists to implicate the susceptibility of nerve roots to compression was that of Gelfan and Tarlov (36). Mechanical compression of the dorsal nerve roots of dogs was accomplished (36):

> The latency of inactivation by pressure, in contrast to the "all-or-nothing" character of the latency of complete anoxia, can be varied over a wide range. It is inversely related to the magnitude of the compressive force and can be graded continuously from intervals of minutes or hours to instantaneous, but reversible, blocking with higher pressures.

Gelfan and Tarlov were in accord with others who had previously acknowledged that larger fibers are more susceptible to compression than are smaller fibers. Since the dorsal spinal root fibers are relatively large, they obviously are clinically important to the chiropractor.

Following up on the work of Gelfan and Tarlov (36), Sharpless (37) utilized a technique that was designed to compress the nerve roots and trunks in graduations, which thus enabled him to determine the minimum pressure needed to achieve a conduction block. A miniature rubber balloon was lowered onto cat and rat nerve roots and trunks. The contact area increased as the pressure applied increased. Thus, at 10 mm Hg an area of 2.5 mm was compressed, and at 50 mm Hg an area of 4.5 mm was constricted. The A components of the action potentials were examined; the astonishing finding was that dorsal spinal roots are far more susceptible to compression than are peripheral nerve trunks (Figure 6.2). The author found that dorsal roots were able to withstand only minimal pressures, as opposed to the sciatic nerves, which were able to withstand far greater pressures. The compound action

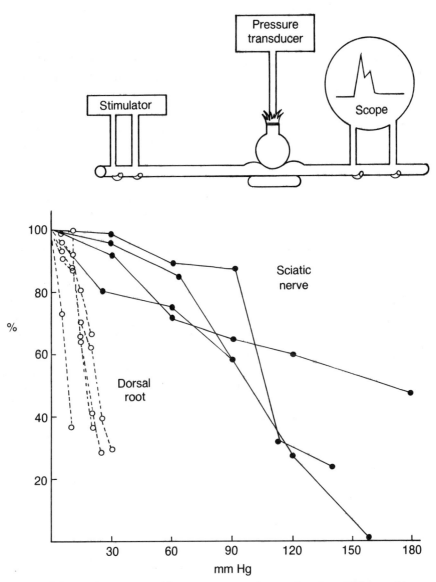

Figure 6.2. Utilizing a variable pressure transducer, Sharpless (37) was able to demonstrate that the A components of the compound action potentials of cat dorsal roots are extremely susceptible to compression block. The compound action potentials (volts x seconds) of the dorsal roots were reduced to half their initial values by a pressure of only 20 mm Hg. By comparison, much greater pressures were necessary in order to similarly affect the sciatic nerve trunks.

potentials (A components) were reduced to about half their initial values at pressures of only 20 to 25 mm Hg. This represents an extraordinary sensitivity to compression. In the case of one rat (some cats had yielded similar results), a pressure of only 10 mm Hg significantly affected conduction such that the compound action potential fell to about 60% of its initial value in only 15 minutes and to 50% of its initial value in just 30 minutes. To illustrate this sensitivity, Sharpless pointed out that the most skilled surgeon could not touch his compression apparatus without recording at least 5 mm Hg. Sharpless believed that this conduction block of some fibers occurred as the result of mechanical deformation rather than hypoxia, or ischemia, since the large fibers are blocked first (anoxia is believed to influence small fibers first). In a recent study, Young and Sharpless (55) found that this sensitivity is altered at the point where the dura forms the epineurium, prior to entry of the roots into the foramina. At this point, the spinal nerves become resistant to compression block.

These findings are in accord with those of MacGregor et al. (27) who, utilizing a pressure vessel model, determined that large fibers would be compressed the most and thus are blocked first (Figure 6.3). It is interesting to note that a pressure vessel model also accounts for the gradient character of nerve root conduction block. The longer that the pressure is applied, the more that viscous displacement occurs in the fibers.

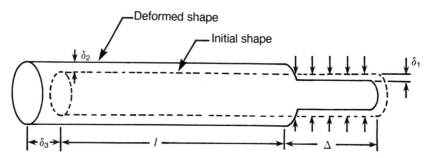

Figure 6.3. MacGregor et al. (27) were able to determine that large nerve fibers should be compressed the most and should be blocked first. According to their model, displaced fluid forces radial distention of the membrane, δ_2, along the length, l, and forces longitudinal displacement, δ_3, at the "end" of the cylinder.

Triano and Luttges (56) were able to demonstrate changes in mouse sciatic nerve consistent with what would be expected in human nerve compression states. Using Silastic plugs affixed adjacent to mouse sciatic nerve *in vivo*, they found a 31% to 40% increase in weight (from accumulation of inflammatory edema) which persisted throughout the test period. Increased nerve weight from edema was responsible for conduction velocity decreases, progressive facilitation in the early (5 to 25 msec) delay periods of nerve refractory sensitivity (by double-pulse studies), and second responses of significantly increased facilitation of refractory recovery that reached maximal levels at 6 days. They believed that such responses to a soft mechanical irritant mimicked neurological disorders faced by the clinician involving minimal nerve irritation or compression, such as sciatic neuritis. Gait disturbances and other behavioral changes in the test mice showed that although gross degenerative changes had not occurred morphologically, some degree of irritation and pain was present.

Luttges and Gerren (57) describe 12 consequences of nerve injury which are not yet fully understood and which include modification of receptor sensitivity, altered fiber projection into the cord, altered sensory input with subsequent changes in cord cells, altered function of Schwann and other supporting cells, sprouting which favors neuromas and single fiber sizes, abnormal reinnervation of tissue due to an appropriate type of nerve, abnormal reinnervation due to an inappropriate type of nerve, afferent neural activity arising from nonreceptor mechanisms, altered axon dimension and temporal patterning of input, sensory fiber activity initiated chemically or electrically by sympathetic afferents, and differential sensory inputs from selective loss of certain fibers or cells. After a comprehensive literature review they concluded that the lack of information regarding nerve root morphology following experimental compression, as well as regarding quantification or characterization of adaptation of dynamic tissue physiology after prolonged compression, has made it difficult at best to corroborate clinical findings with experimental research. Anatomical and physiological considerations of dorsal nerve root and dorsal nerve root ganglion sensitivity to injury include those 12 items cited previously (Figure 6.4).

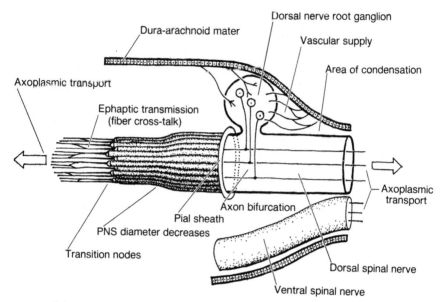

Figure 6.4.   The dorsal nerve root and dorsal nerve root ganglion are susceptible to injury and aberrant function physiologically via a number of mechanisms. This schema illustrates these anatomical and physiological components of dorsal nerve root susceptibility. (Adapted from Luttges MW, Gerren RA: Compression physiology: nerves and roots. In Haldeman S (ed): *Modern Developments in the Principles and Practice in Chiropractic.* New York, Appleton-Century-Crofts, 1980, pp 65–92 (57).)

Various researchers have studied in detail these degenerative and regenerative phenomena and axoplasmic flow and its relationship with nerve crush (25–28). Because axoplasmic flow may be altered by nerve compression, it should be considered as a component of nerve compression pathophysiology. We, however, discuss axoplasmic aberrations in Chapter 10 and regard it as a tertiary hypothesis.

A review of the literature with regard to experimental studies of nerve root and trunk compression thus reveals many findings of great interest to the chiropractic profession and of great importance to chiropractic theory. In summary, compression injuries cause degenerative and regenerative events that result in aberrant levels of certain nerve proteins along the course of the nerve (27–29, 31–37). Although it appears that changes in the velocity and amplitude of the compound action potential occur at the site of compression, the changes in velocity are only temporary (31, 34–

37). The amplitude of the compound action potential, however, appears to be severely and permanently affected by dorsal nerve root compression, although the spinal nerve that exits through the intervertebral foramen is resistant to such compression (36, 37, 55). These effects of nerve root compression appear to be due to biomechanical distortion of the nerve rather than to focal ischemia, as hypothesized by previous authors (31, 35–37).

All-or-None Law

Since the subject of the all-or-none law appears to surface frequently among students and chiropractors, a brief explanation is in order. The all-or-none law refers to the fact, discovered by Bowditch in 1871, that heart muscle—regardless of strength of stimulus—will respond completely or not at all (58, 59). Since that time, studies have confirmed that this principle is valid in other muscles and nerves throughout the body. The law is applicable only to individual nerve fibers, however (58, 59). Gelfan and Tarlov (36) and Sharpless (37) have demonstrated that in studies of nerve compression, block of only some fibers in the nerve is possible. The remaining fibers respond to the stimulus normally (36, 37). Thus, some fibers are blocked while others respond by firing, thereby varying the amplitude of the compound action potential of the nerve. In this way, a subluxation could conceivably affect total nerve output. Hence, there is no disagreement between the all-or-none law and the nerve compression hypothesis.

Clinical Considerations

Nerve root compression of irritation may result in several manifestations that can be clinically confusing to the chiropractor as well as to the orthopedist, neurologist, or specialist in physical medicine (45, 60).

Clinical considerations would include tests to increase the intensity of pain (by coughing, lifting, etc.), which would be indicative of a nerve root compression or lesion (45). Any test that would stretch the involved nerve root (e.g., Lasègue, straight leg raiser, foraminal compression) and produce or intensify pain would also be indicative of a nerve root compression or lesion (45).

Other clinical findings that have been demonstrated in cases of nerve root compression and/or irritation include intermittent claudication with increasing weakness or numbness, leg weakness, sensory changes, limitation of mobility of the involved joint, paravertebral muscle spasm, scoliosis, depressed or absent reflexes in the area of cutaneous innervation, and weakness, paresis, or atrophy of muscles in the involved area of cutaneous innervation (45–47, 54).

Laboratory investigation includes infrared thermography (a positive thermogram is a fairly reliable noninvasive method of evaluating compression nerve injury) and electromyography to determine and differentiate nerve compression (conduction velocity test) from such disorders as descending pathway lesions (H and F reflex tests) (61).

Careful chiropractic analysis is necessary to establish the exact location of the lesion and to determine the correct course of adjustment or other treatment.

Discussion

We may now reach some conclusions, based on this survey of relevant literature, that will help us answer the questions posed earlier in this chapter. There appears to be a significant amount of literature to document the following conclusions:

1. Intervertebral subluxations may cause foraminal encroachment throughout the spine, and especially in the thoracic and lumbar areas (9–18, 38, 39, 46, 47, 49).
2. It is unlikely that neural involvement would occur with thoracic foraminal encroachment (9, 10, 17, 42, 43).
3. It appears probable that some type of traction could expose the highly sensitive nerve roots to the compressive action of the constricted foramen, and it is possible that the roots extend to the intervertebral foramen in some cases (17, 37–40, 49, 62).
4. In many instances, however, the nerve roots combine to form the spinal nerve before they enter the foramen, and the spinal nerve is not very susceptible to compression block but is relatively susceptible to block or derangement of axoplasmic transport (31, 34, 35, 55, 56, 62).

Table 6.1. Summary of pathophysiology of various types of nerve compression

Types of compression	Electrophysiology	Pathophysiology
Mild, brief (37, 64)	Decreased compound action potential, immediate recovery	Demyelination
Mild, chronic (56)	Velocity decreased, facilitation of refractory recovery	Edema
Moderate (31, 34, 65)	Conduction block, recovery takes several weeks	Demyelination
Slow, progressive, chronic (29, 33)		Demyelination
Severe, transient (18, 65)		Proximal edema with fiber disarray; distally, wallerian degeneration
Severe, chronic (66, 67)		Edema; nerves escape perineurium to develop new pathways and/or to remyelinate

5. Nerves affected by foraminal encroachment may undergo degenerative and regenerative processes that impair their function while compressed and until complete regeneration occurs (Table 6.1) (19–22, 25–41, 45–47).

A recent study by Wall et al. (63) confirmed that local pressure applied to the dorsal nerve roots may result in injury discharge lasting up to 18 seconds before conduction block. The many and varied clinical phenomena that have been associated with nerve root involvement are reviewed in this chapter under "Clinical Considerations." Although the data show the distinct possibility that nerve root compression or irritation may result from certain intervertebral subluxations, they do not prove that this relationship is a common clinical entity.

Summary

Palmer (1) proposed the first *nerve compression* hypothesis when he stated that intervertebral subluxations can interfere with the normal transmission of nerve energy. *Subluxation pathophysiology* includes various stages of degenerative and regenerative processes that impair the function of the involved nerve roots, as well as clinical signs and symptoms of intermittent claudication, leg weakness, sensory changes, limitation of mobility of the involved joint, paravertebral muscle spasm, scoliosis, and depressed or absent reflexes in the area of cutaneous innervation (9–22, 25–43, 45–49, 54). The conclusion is reached that although there is a definite possibility that nerve root compression or irritation may be caused by intervertebral subluxations, especially in the cervical and the lumbar spine, it has not been proven that this relationship is a common clinical entity (9–18, 38, 42, 43, 46–49).

References

1. Palmer DD: *The Science, Art and Philosophy of Chiropractic.* Portland, OR, Portland Printing House, 1910.
2. Haldeman S, Drum D: The compression subluxation. *J Clin Chiropractic* (arch ed) 1:10–21, 1971.
3. Hviid H: A consideration of contemporary chiropractic theory. *J Natl Chiropractic Assoc* 25:17–18, 68, 1955.
4. Janse J: Basic concepts of chiropractic theory. In Janse J (ed): *Principles and Practice of Chiropractic.* Lombard, IL, National College of Chiropractic, 1976, pp 43–50.
5. Schreiber T: Neurophysiology triumphant. *J Natl Chiropractic Assoc* 19:21–22, 1949.
6. Schreiber T: Chiropractic—founded on tone. *J Natl Chiropractic Assoc* 19:15–16, 1949.
7. Botta JR (ed): Chiropractors healers or quacks? Part 1: the 80-year war with science. *Consumer Rep* 40(9):542–547, 1975.
8. Crelin ES: A scientific test of the chiropractic theory. *Am Sci* 61:574–580, 1973.
9. Hadley LA: *Anatomico-Roentgenographic Studies of the Spine.* Springfield, IL, Charles C Thomas, 1964, pp 172–183 and 422–477.
10. Hadley LA: Intervertebral joint subluxation, bony impingement and foramen encroachment with nerve root changes. *Am J Rontgenol Rad Ther* 65:377–402, 1951.
11. Braakman R, Penning L: Injuries to the cervical spine. In Vinken PJ, Bruyn GW (eds): *Handbook of Clinical Neurology.* Injuries to the spinal cord part 1. New York, Elsevier, 1976, vol 25, pp 341–345.
12. Epstein JA, Epstein BS, Lavine LS, Carras R, Rosenthal AD, Sumner P: Sciatica caused by nerve root entrapment in the lateral recess: the superior facet syndrome. *J Neurosurg* 36:584–589, 1972.
13. Grogono BJS: Injuries of the atlas and axis. *Br J Bone Joint Surg* 36:397–410, 1954.
14. Chesterman JT: Spontaneous subluxation of the atlantoaxial joint. *Lancet* 1:539, 1936.
15. Schlessinger PT: Incarceration of the 1st sacral nerve in a lateral bony recess of the spinal canal as a cause of sciatica: anatomy—two case reports. *J Bone Joint Surg* 37A:115–124, 1955.
16. Sullivan AW: Subluxation of the atlanto-axial joint. *J Pediatr* 35:451–464, 1949.
17. Sunderland S: Anatomical perivertebral influences on the intervertebral foramen. In Goldstein M (ed): *The Research Status of Spinal Manipulative Therapy.* Washington, DC, Government Printing Office, 1975, pp 129–140.
18. Kovacs A: Subluxation and deformation of the cervical apophyseal joints. *Acta Radiol* 43:1–15, 1955.

19. Lindblom K: Protrusions of discs and nerve compression in the lumbar region. *Acta Radiol* 25:195–212, 1944.
20. Schaumburg HH, Spencer PS: Pathology of spinal root compression. In Goldstein M (ed): *The Research Status of Spinal Manipulative Therapy*. Washington, DC, Government Printing Office, 1975, pp 141–148.
21. Von Reis G: Pain in the distribution area of the 4th lumbar root. *Acta Psychiatr Neurol [Suppl]* 36:1–135, 1945.
22. Frykholm R: Cervical nerve root compression resulting from disc degeneration and root-sleeve fibrosis. *Acta Chir Scand [Suppl]* 160:1–149, 1951.
23. Awad MZ: Induction of intervertebral disrelationship in experimental animals and the preliminary effects of the dysarthrias. In Suh CH (ed): *Proceedings of the 7th Annual Biomechanics Conference on the Spine*. Boulder, CO, University of Colorado, 1976, pp 27–50.
24. Lin H-L, Fujii A, Rebechini-Zasadny H, Hartz DL: Experimental induction of vertebral subluxation in laboratory animals. *J Manip Physiolog Ther* 1:63–66, 1978.
25. Luttges MW, Kelly PT, Gerren RA: Degenerative changes in mouse sciatic nerves: electrophoretic and electrophysiologic characterizations. *Exp Neurol* 50:706–733, 1976.
26. Kelly PT, Luttges MW: Electrophoretic separation of nervous system proteins on exponential gradient polyacrylamide gels. *J Neurochem* 24:1077–1079, 1975.
27. MacGregor RJ, Sharpless SK, Luttges MW: A pressure vessel model for nerve compression. *J Neurol Sci* 24:299–304, 1975.
28. Luttges MW, Groswald DE: Degenerative and regenerative characterizations in the proteins of mouse sciatic nerves. In Suh CH (ed): *Proceedings of the 7th Annual Biomechanics Conference on the Spine*. Boulder Co, University of Colorado, 1976, pp 71–81.
29. Duncan D: Alterations in the structure of nerves caused by restricting their growth with ligatures. *J Neuropathol Exp Neurol* 7:261–273, 1948.
30. Lindblom K, Rexed B: Spinal nerve injury in dorsolateral protrusions of lumbar discs. *J Neurosurg* 5:413–432, 1948.
31. Denny-Brown D, Brenner C: Paralysis of nerve induced by direct pressure and by tourniquet. *Arch Neurol Psychiatr* 51:1–26, 1944.
32. Dyck PJ: Experimental hypertrophic neuropathy. *Arch Neurol* 21:73–95, 1969.
33. Aguayo A, Nair CPV, Midgley R: Experimental progressive compression neuropathy in the rabbit. *Arch Neurol* 24:358–364, 1971.
34. Fowler TJ, Danta G, Gilliatt RW: Recovery of nerve conduction after a pneumatic tourniquet: observations on the hind-limb of the baboon. *J Neurol Neurosurg Psychiatr* 35:638–647, 1972.
35. Rainer GW, Mayer J, Sadler TR, Dirks D: Effect of graded compression on nerve conduction velocity. *Arch Surg* 107:719–721, 1973.
36. Gelfan S, Tarlov IM: Physiology of spinal cord, nerve root and peripheral nerve compression. *Am J Physiol* 185:217–229, 1956.
37. Sharpless SK: Susceptibility of spinal roots to compression block. In Goldstein M (ed): *The Research Status of Spinal Manipulative Therapy*. Washington, DC, Government Printing Office, 1975, pp 155–161.
38. Sunderland S: Mechanisms of cervical nerve root avulsion in injuries of the neck and shoulder. *J Neurosurg* 41:705–714, 1974.
39. Sunderland S, Bradley KC: Stress-strain phenomena in human spinal nerve roots. *Brain* 84:120–124, 1961.
40. Sunderland S: The anatomy of the intervertebral foramen and the mechanisms of compression and stretch of nerve roots. In Haldeman S (ed): *Modern Developments in the Principles and Practice in Chiropractic*. New York, Appleton-Century-Crofts,

1980, pp 45–64.

41. Breig A, Marions O: Biomechanics of the lumbosacral nerve roots. *Acta Radiol* 1:1141–1160, 1962.

42. Hadley LA: Constriction of the intervertebral foramen. *JAMA* 140:473–476, 1949.

43. Hadley LA: Roentgenographic studies of the cervical spine. *Am J Roentgenol* 52:173–195, 1944.

44. Rosomoff HL, Rossman F: Treatment of cervical spondylosis by anterior cervical diskectomy and fusion. *Arch Neurol* 14:392, 1966.

45. Eaton LM: Pain caused by disease involving the sensory nerve roots (root pain). *JAMA* 177:1435–1439, 1941.

46. Epstein JA, Epstein BS, Lavine LS, Carras R, Rosenthal AD, Sumner P: Sciatica caused by nerve root entrapment in the lateral recess: the superior facet syndrome. *J Neurosurg* 36:584–589, 1972.

47. Epstein JA, Epstein BS, Lavine LS, Carras R, Rosenthal AD, Sumner P: Lumbar nerve root compression at the intervertebral foramina caused by arthritis of the posterior facets. *J Neurosurg* 39:362–369, 1973.

48. Triano J, Luttges MW: Subtle, intermittent mechanical irritation of sciatic nerves of mice. In Suh CH (ed): *Proceedings of the 9th Annual Biomechanics Conference on the Spine.* Boulder, CO, University of Colorado, 1978.

49. Sunderland S: Meningeal-neural relations in the intervertebral foramen. *J Neurosurg* 40:756–763, 1974.

50. Drum D: The vertebral motor unit and intervertebral foramen. In Goldstein M (ed): *The Research Status of Spinal Manipulative Therapy.* Washington, DC, Government Printing Office, 1975, pp 63–75.

51. Brain L: Some aspects of neurology of the cervical spine. *J Fac Radiol* 8:74–91, 1956.

52. Olsson Y: Studies on vascular permeability in peripheral nerves, distribution of circulating fluorescent serum albumin in normal, crushed, and sectioned rat sciatic nerve. *Acta Neuropathol* 7:1–15, 1966.

53. Bergmann L, Alexander L: Vascular supply of the spinal ganglia. *Arch Neurol Psychiatr* 46:761–782, 1941.

54. Frykholm R: Deformities of dural pouches and strictures of dural sheaths in the cervical region producing nerve-root compression. *J Neurosurg* 4:403–413, 1947.

55. Young S, Sharpless SK: Mechanisms protecting nerve against compression block. In Suh CH (ed): *Proceedings of the 9th Annual Biomechanics Conference on the Spine.* Boulder CO, University of Colorado, 1978.

56. Triano JJ, Luttges MW: Nerve irritation: a possible model of sciatic neuritis. *Spine* 7:129–136, 1982.

57. Luttges MW, Gerren RA: Compression physiology: nerves and roots. In Haldeman S (ed): *Modern Developments in the Principles and Practice of Chiropractic.* New York, Appleton-Century-Crofts, 1980, pp 65–92.

58. Friel JP (ed): *Dorland's Illustrated Medical Dictionary,* ed 25. Philadelphia, Saunders, 1974, pp 59–60.

59. Guyton AC: *Basic Human Physiology: Normal Function and Mechanisms of Disease.* Philadelphia, Saunders, 1971, pp 54–55.

60. Watkins RJ: Slipped disc? sprain? or syndrome? *Dig Chiropractic Econ* 17:20–23, 1975.

61. Triano JJ: The use of instrumentation and laboratory examination procedures by the chiropractor. In Haldeman S (ed): *Modern Developments in the Principles and Practice of Chiropractic.* New York, Appleton-Century-Crofts, 1980, pp 231–268.

62. Warwick R, Williams PL: *Gray's Anatomy,* British ed 35. Philadelphia, Saunders, 1973.

63. Wall PD, Waxman S, Basbaum AL: Ongoing activity in peripheral nerve: injury discharge. *Exp Neurol* 45:576–589, 1974.

64. Gilliatt RW: The cause of nerve damage in acute compression. *Trans Am Neurol Assoc* 99:71–74, 1974
65. Spinner M, Spencer PS: Nerve compression lesions of the upper extremity. *Clin Orthop* 104:46–67, 1974.
66. Weiss P, Hiscoe HB: Experiments on the mechanism of nerve growth. *J Exp Zool* 107:315–395, 1948.
67. Sunderland S: The effect of rupture of the perineurium on the contained nerve fibres. *Brain* 69:149–152, 1940.

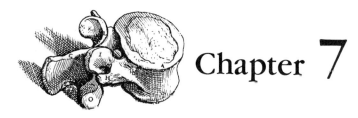

Chapter 7

Cord Compression Hypothesis

*R*elatively little attention in the chiropractic literature has been given to the pathophysiology of spinal cord compression. The founder of chiropractic probably did not think it possible that cord compression could result from subluxations (1). Haldeman (2) in a comprehensive review of the compression subluxation did not mention the possibility of this arthrosis adversely affecting spinal cord function by direct compression. Moreover, in the medical literature it has commonly been reported that fracture/dislocation of vertebrae may result in cord compression; the possibility that severe subluxations could do the same, however, at times has been ignored (3–5). Considerable emphasis was placed on the cord compression mechanism by B. J. Palmer who originated the "hole-in-one" adjustive technique after years of clinical research (6):

> Spinal cord is an accumulation and assembling of all efferent and afferent fibers that go to or come from all the body. As they gather, they more nearly, in ratio, fill neural canal. . . . These facts, plus absence of osseous locking of vertebral motion, make constricted pressure a reality and of paramount and vital importance.

Since Palmer's original observations, a number of medical authors (7–20) have recognized that marked subluxations may play a role in direct compression and displacement of the spinal cord. These investigators have documented case after case in which severe subluxations may (even in the absence of a complicating fracture) cause paresthesias, numbness, transient paraplegia, quadriplegia, and even death. The fascinating and serious finding that crib death or sudden infant death syndrome (SIDS) may be the result of

74

birth trauma and subsequent brain stem involvement after cervical subluxation is reviewed (21–26). In addition to subluxations and fracture/dislocations, spondylosis is recognized as a common cause of spinal cord compression or ischemia when those events occur (27–30). Other causes of cord compression including tumors are briefly discussed in this chapter, along with experimental studies that pertain to this subject (31–37).

Subluxations and Spinal Cord Compression

Various authors (6–15) have reported that severe trauma may cause marked subluxations that compress or otherwise adversely affect the spinal cord. Subluxations associated with arthritides have also been reported to produce brain stem compression (16–20, 38). Lax ligamentous structure has been cited by at least one author as a cause of subluxation that compresses spinal cord structure (8). Nearly all of these cases occur when the articular facets are clearly not overriding (which would be a luxation according to most authors) and there is no evidence of fracture.

These data appear to confirm the hypothesis of Palmer (6) to some degree. His hypothesis was that upper cervical subluxations could cause occlusion of the spinal canal. For the purpose of discussion we will define the *cord compression* hypothesis more broadly; i.e., that intervertebral subluxations may, in some severe cases (and even in the absence of fracture/dislocation), irritate or compress the spinal cord.

In 1911, Ely (11) reported a case in which the atlas was subluxated forward following a 9-ft fall down an elevator shaft. Aside from a cut on the skull, which was dressed, a persistent headache was the only subjective complaint for the next 4 weeks. Shortly thereafter, numbness, tingling, and marked sweating heralded the onset of gradual paralysis of all four extremities, and the patient was admitted to a nearby hospital. On examination, the rectus lateralis and right and left recti postici obliqui superior and inferior muscles were reported to be rigid. Cranial nerve testing was essentially negative. Knee jerks were greatly exaggerated, however, and a positive right Babinski and ankle clonus indicated neurologic dysfunction. It was at this time that on a "skiagram" (x-ray) an atlas-axis subluxation was identified. An exasperating course of treatment followed in which the patient was repeatedly placed in and taken out of plaster cervical collars over a period of months. Each time the collars were applied the objective and subjective findings including paralysis were relieved and remissions ensued. Each time the collars were removed, however, the paralysis returned, to the dismay of patient and doctors alike. Finally, the doctors operated, tying the posterior arches of atlas and axis together, while an anesthesiologist attempted to reduce the subluxation with manipulation, *through the mouth!* Nearly complete paralysis of the limbs, bladder, and rectum immediately followed the operation, but within 3 months the patient was walking again. Six months following the operation, the patient had recovered fully from the subluxation. Without being too facetious, we cannot help but quote one of the doctors involved who summarized the course of treatment by saying, "It is a great case." This was perhaps the first radiographically and operatively documented case of subluxation causing spinal cord compression.

A host of modern neurosurgeons, orthopedists, and radiologists have documented the role subluxation may play in cord compression. Braakman and Penning (7) have identified anterior atlas subluxations as a cause of spinal cord lesions. Guttmann (12) states that spinal cord compression occurs more commonly following subluxation of the cervical spine than of the thoracolumbar spine. Jackson (14), Seletz (19), and Brodsky (9) have recognized the possibility of cord or cauda equina compression following subluxation.

Brain (8) acknowledged that the transverse ligament may become lax, which allows forward atlas subluxation and, with forward flexion of the neck, results in brain stem compression (39).

Osteoarthroses associated with trauma have been identified in the etiology of subluxated lateral facet joints by Brodsky (9).

Following certain accidents, a transient paraplegia (intermittent) and the onset of neurologic signs may be delayed from days to as long as 40 years (9, 14). Hughes (13) acknowledged both operative and postmortem demonstration of subluxations as a cause of spinal cord lesions. He suggested that immediately following a traumatic accident, there may not appear to be any gross abnormality of the spine. Instead, he proposed, a large number of fibers are affected but only to a minor degree (most are recoverable). Jacobson and Adler (15) reported on a case that is in accord with this description. Following an accident, their patient reported loss of sensation in both legs and difficulty in moving all four extremities. Radiologic examination revealed rotational subluxation with probable upper cervical cord compression. An anteroposterior film revealed a 3.5-mm offset of the left articular mass of the atlas. Yet within days, the neurologic and subjective findings disappeared. In the case presented by Jacobson and Adler (15), although there was no delay in onset of neurologic and subjective findings, there was indication that a large number of fibers were slightly affected.

Wollin and Botterell (20) have found neurologic signs indicative of spinal cord involvement in many of their patients with forward dislocations of the atlas on the axis.

In context, it should be mentioned that there is a difference of opinion as to the relative frequency of the subluxation and/or cord lesion. Although some authors have implied or suggested that subluxation and/or cord lesion is a relatively common cause of spinal cord compression (10, 12, 13, 16–18), others have believed that it is rare (19, 39).

One of the syndromes more commonly associated with subluxation and brain stem compression involves the various arthritides. A number of investigators (10, 16–18) have clearly linked subluxations to arthritides; they have believed, however, that the arthritides cause the subluxations. Subsequent spinal cord involvement has been reported by Davidson et al. (10), Rana et al. (16), Matthews (17), and Robinson (18). Rana et al. (16) found atlas-axis subluxation with translocation of the odontoid upward into the medulla oblongata in fully 25% of their patients with rheumatoid arthritis. They determined that the extent of neurologic involvement did not correspond to the degree of subluxation. They noted objective CNS signs and a subsequent narrowing of the spinal canal of 13% to 52% of its normal size in 27 of 41 patients with subluxations. Matthews (17) identified vertical subluxations in 7% of his rheumatoid outpatients. Davidson et al. (10) reported on atlas-axis subluxation causing dysphagia and other neurologic indications in a woman with rheumatoid arthritis. They too found that the subluxation was causing brain stem compression. Robinson (18) suggested that atlas-axis subluxation with subsequent spinal cord compression can lead to development not only of various neurologic signs but also of quadriplegia and even sudden death. He noted the occurrence of occipital headaches, paresthesias, and objective signs of cord compression with sensory and/or pyramidal signs in 14 of 22 patients with atlas-axis subluxation and rheumatoid arthritis. Latchaw and Mayer (38) suggested that subluxation may also be of a frequent occurrence in Reiter's disease (arthritis, nongonococcal urethritis, and conjunctivitis).

Hence, it can be seen that subluxations have been implicated in a wide variety of cases as the direct and indirect cause of brain stem and cord compression (7–18, 38, 39).

Cervical Subluxation with Myelopathy Associated with Sudden Infant Death Syndrome

Sudden infant death syndrome (SIDS) has long been an enigma in pediatric practice. Although current mechanisms and hypotheses suggest that sleep apnea involving chronic or recurring hypoxia is the most likely cause of the great majority of cases of SIDS, a number of other hypotheses have been tested and may be applicable (24–26). The mechanism for sleep apnea is under study and may involve predisposing chemical and anatomical factors; several recognized researchers, however, have identified normal and traumatic birthing as a cause of cervical subluxation with a resultant myelopathy as the underlying cause of a significant number of SIDS cases (21–23).

Alexander et al. (21) reported on a case of atlas subluxation following traumatic birth. In this case, the subluxation was complicated by fracture of the odontoid. Other than initial signs of cerebral palsy, there appeared to be no warning of imminent danger for months after the birth. Yet the infant died following nearly complete paralysis. Postmortem examination revealed that the cord at the first cervical level was one fifth of its normal size (Figure 7.1). The authors believed that had the displacement been identified even 1 month prior to death, surgical intervention could have restored the cord to near-normal function.

Schmorl and Junghanns (22) reviewed European medical research regarding SIDS and cervical spine injury. Noting that there was increased incidence of disruption of the spine especially with breech deliveries, the authors concluded that subarachnoid hemorrhage, hematomyelia, and cervical subluxation are frequently observed (22):

> Even very severe injuries of the spinal cord have occurred without demonstrable spinal damage. In the case of forceps deliveries, spinal

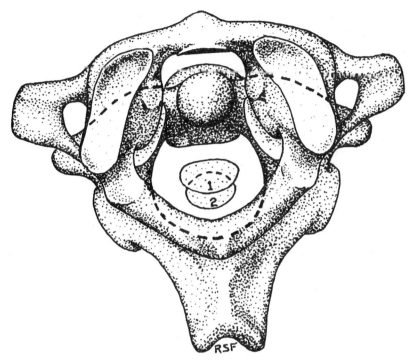

Figure 7.1. Schematic diagram of superior view of the atlas-axis shows subluxation of the atlas anteriorly, with resultant flattening of the spinal cord (*1*) at the first cervical level. According to Schmorl and Junghanns (22), even normal deliveries can result in injuries to the upper area of the cervical spine of the newborn.

cord damages are found predominantly along the cervicothoracic transition. Normal deliveries are frequently associated with injuries to the upper area of the cervical spine. Therefore, [the] possibility of distortions and subluxations of the skull articulations should be kept in mind.

In reviewing his classical work on the subject of SIDS and neonatal injury, Towbin (23) found spinal cord injury in 30 of 170 cases and varying degrees of brain stem injury in 13 of 430 cases. He cited an extensive review of the literature which indicated that significant spinal cord or brain stem injury was found in 10% to 33% of cases of neonatal death at autopsy. In Towbin's study, prior difficulties of histological preparation of the friable newborn brain stem were overcome by use of the technique of whole brain embedding and serial histological sectioning of the brain. Towbin was able to group neonatal deaths from spinal cord or brain stem injury into three classifications: deaths occurring at or shortly after birth due to intolerable stress or injury to brain stem or cord structures; deaths occurring several days after birth in patients whose cardiac function is strong but in whom respiratory depression is seen at birth and is later complicated by pneumonia or hyaline membrane disease; and deaths occurring in infants who may live for months or years but in whom may be found initial significant reversible or persistent neurological defects as the only signs of imminent danger. Towbin (23) concluded that

> . . . there must exist a large number of instances with mild injury, with minimal neurologic symptoms, going unnoticed clinically or being relegated to the category of cerebral palsy.

Towbin suggested that the cerebral hypoxic damage found after many brain stem and cord injuries leads to widespread neuronal devastation, especially in the forebrain; cerebral palsy, mental retardation, epilepsy, and other nervous system disorders may be the ultimate result.

The role of spinal cord and brain stem injury in causing hypoxia and eventually resulting in crib death has been enhanced by current research on SIDS. Hence, in a recent exhaustive review of literally hundreds of SIDS research projects worldwide, Valdes-Dapena (24) concluded that hypoventilation and altered cardiac function are significant risks for near-miss infants, since these conditions predispose infants to sudden death. Analyzing conclusions reached by researchers of other hypotheses regarding etiology of SIDS (including prolonged Q-T interval, viral infection, botulism, postmortem vitreous humor, toxic agents, thiamine metabolism, infanticide, allergic response to house dust mites, and DPT immunizations), she found evidence that could explain only a few causes of SIDS. Considerable weight, however, was placed on the findings that tissue markers for hypoxia and hypoxemia have been identified in SIDS victims at postmortem examination. As a group, SIDS infants are morphologically different from normal infants at autopsy. Hence, chronic hypoxia (hypoventilation) resulted in increased medial muscle mass in walls of small pulmonary arteries and in increased weight of the right cardiac ventricle, while chronic hypoxemia resulted in, among other things, abnormal gliosis in the respiratory centers of the brain stem. An interesting anatomical variation found in one study indicated that the posterior arch of the atlas in 10 of 17 infants inverted through the foramen magnum on extension of the head, which resulted in the potential for bilateral vertebral artery compression (and brain stem hypoperfusion which leads to SIDS).

More recent research has continued to support a hypoxia mechanism for SIDS. Kahn and Blum (25) have rejected the hypothesis that SIDS is the result of overheating and an abnormal thermoregulatory system. Kinney et al. (26) have reaffirmed the finding of brain stem gliosis after chronic hypoxemia. In five areas of the medulla oblongata which are related to involuntary respiration, significantly more reactive astrocytes were found at postmortem examination in SIDS victims than in normal infants. This finding, of course, lends support to the theory that there is a mechanism of SIDS which involves a sleep apnea and which is precipitated by defective control of involuntary respiration.

Although it is not yet known how significant a role spinal cord and brain stem injury with subluxation may play in causing the hypoxia or chronic hypoxemia that leads to crib death, there is strong evidence from the literature to suggest such a role in a significant number of cases (21–26).

Spondylosis and Spinal Cord Compression

It is widely accepted that spondylosis with its degenerative and arthritic events can lead to spinal cord compression (27–30). Several authors (27–29) have implicated osteophytic bars growing out from the ventral wall of the spinal canal as the mechanism for compression in cases of spondylosis of the cervical vertebrae. Gooding (30) has provided a more elaborate mechanism that may explain cord involvement and the neurologic signs that are noted. He proposes that the spondylotic degenerative events produce spinal nerve root fibrosis and that this fibrosis induces a general spasm of the lateral spinal arteries, which subsequently produces spinal cord ischemia in the cervical region. Interestingly, spondylosis is associated with subluxations in many instances by some authors (27, 28).

Experimental Studies of Spinal Cord Compression

Studies by several researchers tend to support the Gooding (30) concept that the spinal nerves may play an important role in production of cervical cord symptoms. For instance, Hukuda and

Wilson (31) in experiments on the spinal cords of dogs determined that the effects of vascular insufficiency and mechanical compression are additive. Hence, even a slight degree of nerve root fibrosis, when combined with osteophytic growth in the spinal canal, could result in changes sufficient to produce subjective and objective findings. In another interesting study, Tarlov and Klinger (32) found that light compression of the canine spinal cord for 15 to 120 minutes resulted in instantaneous sensory/motor paralysis which was completely reversible. In further studies, Gelfan and Tarlov (33) determined that dorsal column fibers were the most sensitive to mechanical compression and were the slowest to recover after the pressure was released.

Other Etiologies of Spinal Cord Compression

Besides the more common causes of spinal cord compression—fracture/dislocations, subluxations, and osteophytes and ischemia associated with spondylosis—there are some lesser known clinical entities. Tumors, although rare, are obviously given attention (34–36). Boyd (34) classifies spinal cord tumors as either extramedullary or intramedullary. Extramedullary tumors are frequently benign and are of two types: extradural, which is the more severe and is commonly a metastatic carcinoma or lymphoma; and intradural, which is the more common, is usually benign, and may persist for some time before signs of cord or nerve root involvement appear. Although the cord may be severely compressed by a tumor, it still has a remarkable ability to recover (34). Hence, operative removal of the lesion often may result in positive recovery (34). In addition to tumors, other lesions have been associated with spinal cord compression. In one report, a case of spastic paraplegia appeared to have been caused by an extradural mass of lipid that was found to be symmetrically compressing the subarachnoid space and the cord (37). Yet operatively, it was seen that the cord compression was due instead to dural constriction that had completely obliterated the subarachnoid space and shut off the flow of cerebrospinal fluid. This lesion was associated with the juvenile onset of diabetes mellitus, according to these authors (37). (For discussion on differentiating spinal cord and other lesions, consult the appendix.)

Discussion

It seems most likely that a combination of factors results in spinal cord compression or insufficiency. It is known that subluxations can affect the second cervical nerve adversely, and by the pathway described by Gooding (30) the resultant spasm of spinal arteries could conceivably render the cord ischemic (6, 19). This would selectively block multisynaptic responses first, according to the research of some investigators (33). In addition, more severe subluxations—especially with upward translocation of the odontoid—have been demonstrated as a direct cause of cord compression (7, 8, 10–18). Mechanical compression appears to affect the dorsal column fibers (kinesthetic sensations, fine pressure, fine touch, and vibratory sense) more quickly and for longer duration (longer recovery time necessary) than do other fibers (33). Spondylotic events commonly occur with subluxations, and it is all too conceivable to envision that osteophytes could combine with less severe subluxations to produce mechanical cord compression in many unrecognized, subclinical cases (27–30).

Similarly, anatomical and physiological variations in the cervical spine of the neonate may predispose it to the traction and extension forces used during even normal delivery to cause subluxation, brain stem or cord damage, chronic hypoxia or hypoxemia, and crib death (21–26). Even adults with low anteroposterior diameters of the spinal canal have significantly increased myelopathy after trauma (40). Hence, anatomical and physiological variance plays an important role in the development of myelopathy. What role subluxation of the apophyseal joints may play remains to be fully explored, but it is suggested that myelopathy after subluxation may be more likely if the spine is anatomically or physiologically predisposed to such an event.

Summary

Severe subluxations have been demonstrated as a cause of spinal cord compression (7, 8, 10–18). Cervical spine injury and, specifically, subluxation have been associated with brain stem and cord injury that leads to hypoxia, hypoxemia, and crib death (SIDS) even after "normal" delivery (21–26). This finding is consistent with the cord compression hypothesis. Spondylosis, fracture/dislocations, and tumors have also been documented as etiologies of cord insufficiency and/or compression (3–5, 27–30, 34–36). Experimental research indicates that the effects of these lesions could be additive (31). Possible effects of cord compression include headache, numbness, tingling, paresthesias, quadriplegia, transient paraplegia, practically any combination of neurologic findings, and even death (7, 10, 11, 13, 15, 16–19).

References

1. Palmer DD: *The Science, Art and Philosophy of Chiropractic.* Portland, OR, Portland Printing House, 1910.
2. Haldeman S: The compression subluxation. *J. Clin Chiropractic* (arch ed) 1:10–21, 1971.
3. Frank I: Spontaneous (nontraumatic) atlanto-axial subluxation. *Ann Otol Rhinol Laryngol* 45:405–411, 1936.
4. Vick N: *Grinker's Neurology,* ed 7. Springfield, IL, Charles C Thomas, 1976.
5. Eliasson SG, et al: *Neurological Pathophysiology.* New York, Oxford University Press, 1974.
6. Palmer BJ: *The Subluxation Specific—The Adjustment Specific.* Davenport, IA, Palmer School of Chiropractic, 1934, p 205.
7. Braakman R, Penning L: Injuries to the cervical spine. In Vinken PJ, Bruyn GW (eds): *Handbook of Clinical Neurology.* Injuries to the spinal cord part 1. New York, Elsevier, 1976, vol 25, pp 341–345.
8. Brain R: Some aspects of the neurology of the cervical spine. *J Fac Radiol* 8:74–91, 1956.
9. Brodsky AE: Low back pain syndromes due to spinal stenosis and posterior cauda equina compression. *Bull Hosp Joint Dis* 36:66–79, 1975.
10. Davidson RC, Horn JR, Herndon JH, Grin OD: Brain stem compression in rheumatoid arthritis. *JAMA* 238:2633–2634, 1977.
11. Ely LW: Subluxation of the atlas, *Ann Surg* 54:20–29, 1911.
12. Guttman L: Conservative management. In Vinken PJ, Bruyn GW (eds): *Handbook of Clinical Neurology.* Injuries to the spinal cord part 2. New York, Elsevier, 1976, vol 26, pp 289–306.
13. Hughes JT: Spinal cord trauma. In: *Greenfield's Neuropathology.* London, Edward Arnold, 1976, pp 665–666.
14. Jackson R: *The Cervical Syndrome.* Springfield, IL, Charles C Thomas, 1978.
15. Jacobson G, Adler DC: Examination of the atlanto-axial joint following injury. *Am J Roentgenol* 76:1081–1094, 1956.
16. Rana NA, Hancock DO, Taylor AR, Hill AGS: Atlanto-axial subluxation and upward translocation of the odontoid process in rheumatoid arthritis. *Am J Bone Joint Surg* 55A:1304, 1973.
17. Matthews JA: Atlanto-axial subluxation in rheumatoid arthritis: a five-year follow-up study. *Ann Rheum Dis* 33:526–531, 1974.
18. Robinson HS: Rheumatoid arthritis—atlanto-axial subluxation and its clinical presentation. *Can Med Assoc J* 94:470–477, 1966.
19. Seletz E: Trauma and the cervical portion of the spine. *J Int Col Surg* 40:47–62, 1963.
20. Wollin DG, Botterell FH: Symmetrical forward luxation of the atlas. *Am J Roentgenol* 79:575–583, 1958.
21. Alexander E, Masland R, Harris C: Anterior dislocation of first cervical vertebra simulating cerebral birth injury in infancy. *Am J Dis Child* 85:173–181, 1953.

22. Schmorl G, Junghanns H: *Human Spine in Health and Disease*, ed 2. New York, Grune & Stratton, 1972, p 272.

23. Towbin A: Latent spinal cord and brain stem injury in newborn infants. *Dev Med Child Neurol* 11:54–68, 1969.

24. Valdes-Dapena MA: Sudden infant death syndrome: a review of the medical literature 1974–1979. *Pediatrics* 66:597–614, 1980.

25. Kahn A, Blum D: Letter to the editor (in reply). *Pediatrics* 71:987, 1983.

26. Kinney HC, Burger PC, Harrell FE, Hudson RP: 'Reactive gliosis' in the medulla oblongata of victims of the sudden infant death syndrome. *Pediatrics* 72:181–187, 1983.

27. Sandler B: Cervical spondylosis as a cause of spinal cord pathology. *Arch Phys Med Rehabil* 42:650–659, 1961.

28. Crandall PH, Batzdorf U: Cervical spondylotic myelopathy. *J Neurosurg* 25:57–66, 1966.

29. Breig A, Turnbull I, Hassler D: Effects of mechanical stresses on the spinal cord in cervical spondylosis. *J Neurosurg* 25:45–56, 1966.

30. Gooding MR: Pathogenesis of myelopathy in cervical spondylosis. *Lancet* 2:1180–1181, 1974.

31. Hukuda S, Wilson CB: Experimental cervical myelopathy: effects of compression and ischemia on the canine cervical cord. *J Neurosurg* 37:631–652, 1972.

32. Tarlov IM, Klinger H: *Arch Neurol Psychiatr* 71:271, 1954.

33. Gelfan S, Tarlov IM: Physiology of spinal cord, nerve root and peripheral nerve compression. *Am J Physiol* 185:217–229, 1956.

34. Boyd W: *A Textbook of Pathology*, ed 8. Philadelphia, Lea & Febiger, 1970, pp 1281–1282.

35. Meschan I: *Synopsis of Analysis of Roentgen Signs in General Radiology*. Philadelphia, Saunders, 1976, p 623.

36. Berkow R (ed): *The Merck Manual*, ed 14. Rahway, NJ, Merck & Co, 1982, pp 1352–1353.

37. Heilbrun MP, Davis DO: Spastic paraplegia secondary to cord constriction by the dura. *J Neurosurg* 39:645–647, 1973.

38. Latchaw RE, Mayer GW: Reiter disease with atlantoaxial subluxation. *Radiology* 126:303–304, 1978.

39. Hess JH, Bronstein IP, Abelson SM: Atlanto-axial dislocation. *Am J Dis Child* 49:1137–1147, 1935.

40. Epstein N, Epstein JA, Benjamin V, Ransohoff J: Traumatic myelopathy in patients with cervical spinal stenosis without fracture or dislocation; methods of diagnosis, management, and prognosis. *Spine* 5:489–496, 1980.

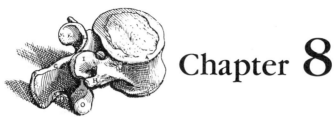

Chapter 8

Fixation Hypothesis

*F*ollowing the lead of Junghanns (1), those chiropractors, osteopaths, and medical doctors who specialize in manipulation have generally come to recognize spinal "fixation" (SF) as a vertebral motor unit that has lessened mobility (2–5). It is acknowledged by these specialists that in these patients the vertebra(e) is (are) "locked" within its (their) normal range of motion. Some chiropractors and osteopaths, however, have hypothesized further that this "fixation" can create the noxious or nociceptive input necessary to trigger abnormal somatosomatic and somatoautonomic reflexes as well as pain (6–9). Some researchers have implied that this SF hypothesis, if proven, could offer the most reasonable explanation for utilizing manipulation in the treatment of conditions other than pain syndromes (10–11), especially since evidence presented at the most recent interdisciplinary manipulation conferences is clear on this point. Nociceptive and somatic afferent bombardment of the dorsal horns of the spinal cord can indeed affect the autonomic nervous system and to some degree affect visceral functions (see Chapter 11). Several important questions must be addressed in order to validate or reject this hypothesis: Has a SF been proven to occur? If it has, will it trigger abnormal or noxious impulse traffic? Will this input be sufficient to initiate or alter somatosomatic and somatoautonomic reflexes, and to what degree?

Although Verner (6), Hviid (9), and others in chiropractic have long held that proprioceptive or nociceptive input from spinal structures could cause functional disorders, the exact origin of the hypothesis remains unknown. Some have suggested that osteopathic researchers were the first to identify the SF (M. Gatterman, personal communication). Homewood (8) dealt with the SF hypothesis in some detail in his book, *The Neurodynamics of the*

Vertebral Subluxation. Haldeman (12, 13) has discussed the evidence relating to such a hypothesis and has detailed some major spinal and paraspinal pathways that would be involved. In order to clarify the hypothesis, we will restate its principal components:

1. *Fixation*—the vertebra is in normal or abnormal position but is "fixed" within its normal range of motion. (See also Table 3.1.)
2. *Soft tissue*—paraspinal musculature and kinesthetic receptors are involved.
3. *Nociceptive or aberrant output*—there is somatic afferent bombardment of spinal pathways.
4. *Segmental facilitation*—is created by afferent bombardment that can affect normal somatic and autonomic reflex traffic.

Hence, the *fixation* hypothesis holds that one type of subluxation is recognized by lessened mobility, soft tissue involvement, aberrant neural reflexes, and segmental facilitation. This hypothesis thus suggests that the effects of the SF may include alteration of neural activity.

In this chapter, we describe in some detail what is known about the SF in terms of clinical and experimental evidence. The neuroanatomy and neurophysiology of the mechanoreceptors involved in proprioception and kinesthetics are reviewed. Spinal pathways that would be involved in transfer of noxious or nociceptive impulses to higher neural centers are described, and the possibility that these impulses affect normal autonomic and somatic function is weighed. In addition, the Korr model of SF is described and discussed.

Clinical Evidence of Spinal Fixation

Until the concept of the vertebral motor unit was synthesized by Junghanns (1), chiropractors to a large degree regarded chiropractic adjustment as a technique for moving a bone that was "out of place" "back into place." This view generally regarded the role of joint mobility as relatively unimportant. Junghanns, however, arranged the spine according to vertebral motor units or "motion segments" in which the soft-tissue components played an important role. In Junghanns' model, the articular facets determine the direction of movement of adjacent vertebrae according to their angles of inclination. Chiropractors and others in the manipulative field have devised, based on Junghanns' model, techniques that emphasize increasing joint mobility when it has been restricted (14–17). This restriction of joint motion is termed a "fixation" by these clinicians, and until recently, this clinical phenomenon has been largely unexplored.

Perhaps osteopathic researchers were the first to begin to explore the possibility of fixations. At any rate, Denslow and Hassett (18) studied *muscle spasm* (i.e., skeletal muscle that displays some degree of rigidity, is tender, and is resistant to pressure deformation) in individuals that had been shown to have postural abnormalities. Electromyographic (EMG) recordings were made of the spinal extensors (glutei, tibialis anterior, and extensor digitorum longus) in subjects lying prone with the head in midline. Sometimes, when electrodes were placed for 1 to 45 minutes, no activity would be recorded; it was suggested that these muscles were in the normal resting state, as confirmed in other EMG studies.

In other muscles, spontaneous activity could be demonstrated without aparent cause (18). These latter muscles were labeled "lesions" by these osteopathic researchers. Utilizing pricking and needle scratching stimuli as well as the application of direct pressure or ice, these scientists were able to demonstrate that these noxious stimuli evoked EMG activity 72.7% of the time (based on 55 applications) in lesioned areas, and only 0.9% of the time in control muscles. When activity was evoked in the control muscles by the stimuli, it was always transient. In contrast, activity evoked in the lesion areas persisted for relatively long periods of time (up to 10 minutes). As further evidence of the phenomenon, two subjects with no obvious symptoms of neuromuscular lesions were used as controls. Ten applications of noxious stimuli in these individuals yielded only minor activity once. The authors believed that the activity demonstrated in lesioned areas could be used as an indirect indicator of afferent bombardment of the spinal cord. They hypothesized that the additional activity evoked from the "lesioned" areas could be explained by Sherrington's concept that subthreshold stimuli (such as were used in their experiments) can create an enduring subliminal *central excitatory state* (CES) in a motoneuron pool. They noted that the CES was seen in lesioned areas in supposedly healthy individuals.

In another examination of the CES, Denslow (19) studied the effects of pressure stimuli applied to the spinous processes of human subjects. It is noteworthy that EMG analysis revealed slight but significantly increased mean thresholds for reflex muscle contraction on the left side rather than on the right side of spinous processes in human subjects. The analysis revealed also that wide differences between thresholds in different individuals and between thresholds at different segmental levels in the same individual are common. Recordings taken at the same segmental level in the same individual on different days, however, showed a relative constancy. The differences noted were attributed to a) changes in the environment of deep pressure or stretch receptors (in medium- and high-threshold areas) and to changes in free nerve endings (in low-threshold zones) and b) an imbalance of excitor-inhibitor influences (e.g., enduring subliminal CES). Denslow et al. (20) concluded that low-threshold segments are in a state of facilitation due to chronic bombardment of impulses from an unknown source. In their studies, the motor reflex threshold correlated to pain thresholds, to susceptibility of supraspinous tissues to minor trauma, and to tissue texture. They suggested that there was an implication that neurons other than the motoneurons in the low-threshold segments might be simultaneously facilitated.

In addition to these clinical investigations of muscle spasm or "lesion" phenomena, clinicians have described and investigated the phenomena of "weakened" and "tight" muscles by use of EMG recordings of muscles contracted in opposition to measured external forces (21, 22). Lewit (23) has investigated the relationship of muscle spasm to the phenomenon of joint fixation; his conclusions vary from the Korr model of SF (to be presented) in that Lewit identifies the joint articulation as the principal "fixation" factor.

Although others have studied this problem, research in this area has been scanty (10). The clinical empirical data collected by chiropractic, osteopathic, and other researchers in this field suggest that phenomena which may be seen and felt in the area of "somatic dysfunction" may be divided into three basic groups:

1. Asymmetry and structural and functional disrelationships, including postural deviations (24, 25).
2. Increased, decreased, or otherwise abnormal joint motion (23–25).
3. Neurologic phenomena which include tissue texture abnormalities as evidenced visually and by light and deep palpation (i.e., changes in color, temperature, and consistency). Muscles in spasm have been described as tender, resistant to pressure deformation, and typically an area displaying some sort of rigidity (18, 24, 25).

Manipulation has been demonstrated to be successful in eliminating the spontaneous localized motor unit activity seen in areas of paraspinal muscle spasm (26, 27). EMG readings following active mobilization of the adjacent vertebrae were shown to be void of the spontaneous potentials noted prior to the manipulation (26, 27).

Thus, it has been established that spinal fixation (SF) does occur and does trigger abnormal or noxious impulses. Before it is possible to answer the last of the three questions originally asked, Will this input be sufficient to initiate or alter somatosomatic and somatoautonomic reflexes, and to what degree?, a basic review of neuromuscular anatomy and physiology as well as of the principal spinal pathways that would mediate such noxious reflexes is in order.

Neurobiology of Kinesthetic Receptors

Several receptors signal the nervous system concerning position and inclination of the joints of the spinal column. These joint receptors together with the various muscle receptors, which report the tension of the skeletal muscles, must play an important role in any afferent bombardment that may accompany the SF (11–13).

The joint receptors include the complex nerve endings, free nerve endings, and Vater-Pacini corpuscles. Of the complex nerve endings, the spray or Ruffini-type endings are the most common within the joint capsules and nearby ligaments. These endings, which are supplied by Type A beta afferents (Table 8.1), are

Table 8.1. Properties of various mammalian nerve fibers[a]

Fiber type	Diameter (μm)	Velocity (m sec)	Function
A (α)	13–22	70–120	Motor, proprioception; sensory transmission of nociception
(β)	8–13	30–70	Touch, kinesthesia
(γ)	4–8	15–40	Motor, spindle excitation; touch, pressure
(δ)	1–5	5–30	Nociceptive reflexes, heat, cold, pressure
B	1–3	3–15	Preganglionic autonomic
C	0.2–1.3	0.2–2.3	Pain (possibly heat, cold, pressure), postganglionic autonomic

[a] Adapted from various sources (28, 31–33).

sensitive to stretch and intra-articular pressure changes and indicate movement and position (28–31). Another joint receptor sensitive to stretch and intra-articular pressure change is the Golgi tendon-type receptor sometimes found in ligaments near the joint. Simple coiled end organs are found in the adventitia of blood vessels and represent the third type of complex nerve endings.

Free nerve endings are found in articular capsule blood vessels, synovial membrane, and external parts of the collateral ligaments. Nociceptive (pain) receptors that are, by nature, these free nerve endings are supplied by unmyelinated and small myelinated fibers. Another type of free nerve ending is the sinuvertebral nerve; its endings provide the fascia, ligaments, periosteum, intervertebral joints, and intervertebral disc with an afferent supply (28–31).

Vater-Pacini corpuscles are not found in the synovial membrane but are sometimes seen in the intervertebral joints; these corpuscles, which are stimulated by movements that distort their lamellar endings, are highly sensitive yet rapidly adapting receptors (28–31).

The muscle receptors play a central role in the Korr model of SF, which is presented later in this chapter. Muscle receptors include the muscle spindle receptors, Golgi tendon organs, pressure receptors, and unmyelinated pain receptors. The function of these receptors is understood in some detail by neurophysiologists (12, 28–31, 34, 35).

The muscle spindle (Figure 8.1) consists of three to ten intrafusal muscle fibers that are pointed at their ends and attach to the sheaths of the surrounding extrafusal (skeletal muscle) fibers. The heavily nucleated central region of the intrafusal fiber cannot contract but can be stretched when surrounding muscle is stretched or when the ends of the intrafusal fibers are contracted. Encompassing the central region is the primary (i.e., annulospiral) receptor which is supplied by a large Type A afferent nerve fiber. A secondary receptor in the muscle spindle is the flower-spray receptor which lies between the annulospiral receptor and the contractile portion of the intrafusal fiber on both sides. The intrafusal fiber itself receives its efferent innervation from Type A gamma motoneurons (fusimotor). The surrounding extrafusal muscle fibers are supplied by large Type A alpha motoneurons (skeletomotor).

Stretch of the muscle belly results in stretch of the intrafusal fibers and activation of the annulospiral endings. The large Type A alpha afferent nerve fibers of the annulospiral receptor synapse directly on Type A alpha motoneurons in the anterior horn of the spinal column. Hence, when the annulospiral endings are activated, reflex contraction of the extrafusal fibers of the same muscle belly occurs. This contraction, in turn, shortens the intrafusal fibers and stops the annulospiral excitation, which allows the muscle to relax. Because this entire mechanism is mediated at a spinal level, it is called a SERVO mechanism. This mechanism of reflex contraction is called the "stretch reflex" (i.e., myotatic reflex) and serves to protect the muscle from stretch beyond its desired length. The annulospiral receptors also are activated on contraction of the intrafusal muscle fibers which contract the two ends of the spindle while stretching the middle.

One important difference between the primary and the secondary muscle spindle receptors is in their phasic responses. The annulospiral endings are more sensitive to changes in intrafusal fiber length and respond faster than the secondary flower-spray receptors. At maximum physiologic length, however, the secondary receptors discharge at higher rates than do the primary receptors. During the resting state the primary receptors enjoy a basal level of activity while the flower-spray endings are inactive.

There is some degree of overlap with regard to fusimotor

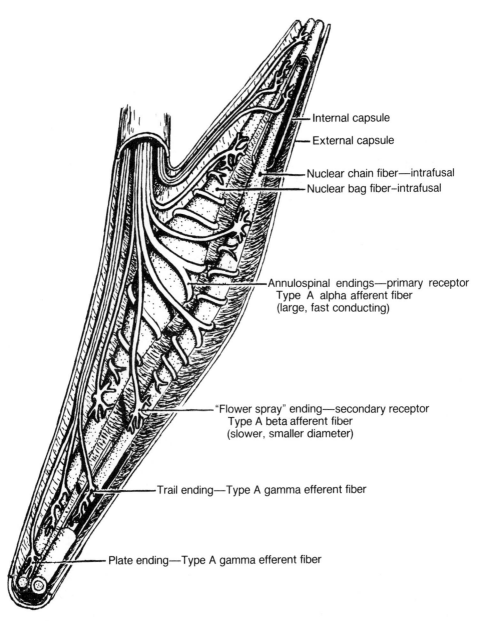

Internal capsule

External capsule

Nuclear chain fiber—intrafusal
Nuclear bag fiber–intrafusal

Annulospinal endings—primary receptor
Type A alpha afferent fiber
(large, fast conducting)

"Flower spray" ending—secondary receptor
Type A beta afferent fiber
(slower, smaller diameter)

Trail ending—Type A gamma efferent fiber

Plate ending—Type A gamma efferent fiber

Figure 8.1. Illustration of the muscle spindle. Two types of intrafusal fibers as well as the annulospiral and flower spray receptors are shown. An external capsule surrounds the entire muscle spindle. The muscle spindle is an important component of the Korr hypothesis of SF. (Adapted from Warwick R, Williams PL (eds): *Gray's Anatomy*, ed 35. Philadelphia, Saunders, 1973, p 800 (30).)

(gamma motoneuron) and skeletomotor (alpha motoneuron) activity. Burke et al. (36) suggest that fusimotor activation during skeletomotor activation provides background discharge for the spindle endings such that they are able to detect irregularities in movement and reflexly correct these irregularities.

The Golgi tendon organ is another muscle receptor that receives its afferent supply from large Type A nerve fibers. This organ consists of receptor endings in a tendon that is attached to 10 to 15 extrafusal muscle fibers; this receptor is stimulated by tension produced in these fibers or by passive stretch of the muscle tendon.

Two types of pressure receptors are also found in skeletal muscle. Regular free nerve endings are the most common pressure-sensitive receptors found in extrafusal muscle. These Type A delta fibers also convey nociceptive as well as thermal sensations at relatively low rates of conduction. Perhaps the most familiar pressure receptor located in muscular tissues is the pacinian corpuscle. This organ is located mainly in the fascia surrounding skeletal muscle fibers. The pacinian receptor consists of concentric lamellae with an unmyelinated nerve ending. The myelinated afferent supply to the pacinian corpuscle transmits impulses for rapid mechanical deformation but no stretch.

Unmyelinated pain receptors comprise another category of muscle receptors. These free branching nerve endings are activated by ischemia, pressure, and thermal changes. These receptors are the terminal endings of the perivascular nerves.

Spinal Pathways and Noxious Stimuli

The central nervous system (CNS) may be thought of as a system of literally hundreds of *neuronal pools*, some of which are very large (e.g., cerebral cortex) (28). Many afferent and efferent fiber tracts as well as interconnecting neurons can be found within any given pool. Apparently, it is this network that allows the nervous system to instantaneously and selectively process the billions of data it is fed every minute. In this way, the CNS can decide which information is important and which should be "ignored" (28).

Both the lateral fibers of the spinothalamic system and the medial fibers of the dorsal column system can be affected by the phenomena of facilitation, inhibition, convergence, divergence, synaptic after discharge, and synaptic fatigue (28). Both of these fiber tracts may be considered as individual neuronal pools.

As with other neuronal pools, these tracts may contain an unknown number of reverberating circuits that add to the effect of *synaptic afterdischarge* (a postsynaptic potential develops in the neuron after discharge, and for many milliseconds a sustained signal output ensues. This discharge lasts for up to 15 msec in anterior motoneurons) (28). Generally, either temporal or spatial summation (or both) must occur before excitation threshold is reached. Subthreshold activity creates a state of facilitation in which the neuron is in "readiness" to begin discharging. Summation may occur in which more than one excitatory postsynaptic potential reaches the same neuron within 15 msec either from the same presynaptic terminal (temporal summation) or from several presynaptic terminals. A neuron that is maximally summated discharges up to 1000 or more times/sec, while one that is barely summated may discharge 15 to 20 impulses/sec. In neurophysiology these and other basic concepts are needed for an understanding of how noxious stimuli may affect spinal pathways and normal neural transmission.

All somatic sensations of a mechanoreceptive or a proprioceptive nature must first enter the dorsal horn of the spinal column before proceeding to other higher neural centers. Holloway et al. (37) found that the phenomenon of *descending inhibition* can affect neural transmission in the dorsal horn cells. These cells may be inhibited by primary afferent depolarization (PAD) which gives rise to presynaptic inhibition of transmission at the interneuron level. The caudal reticular formation, lateral reticular formation, midbrain periaqueductal gray, and medial vestibular nucleus have been shown to be functional in powerful suppression of dorsal horn responses to nociceptive and nonnoxious stimuli (37–39). That there are functionally different midbrain controls of descending inhibition has also now been demonstrated (38, 39). Thus, whether or not pain impulses will be permitted to pass from primary to second order neurons is determined by a complex interaction of neural pathways and neurotransmitters (5-hydroxytryptamine is a direct inhibitor; substance P causes the release of endorphins; glutamate and encephalin are also thought to participate in inhibition) (40) (Figure 8.2).

Another type of neural inhibition involves the role of the sub-

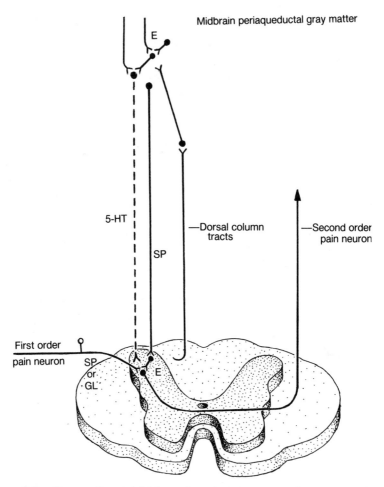

Figure 8.2. Descending inhibition of nociception arises from midbrain peri-aqueductal gray, the caudal reticular formation, the lateral reticular formation, and the medial vestibular nucleus (the latter three are not shown in this schema). These controls are functionally different, and through a complex interaction in which substance P (*SP*), encephalin (*E*), 5-hydroxytryptamine (*5-HT*), and glutamate (*GL*) are utilized as inhibitory neurotransmitters, these brain centers can markedly affect transmission of nociception. (Adapted from Haldeman S: Neurophysiology of spinal pain syndromes. In Haldeman S (ed): *Modern Developments in the Principles and Practice of Chiropractic*. New York, Appleton-Century-Crofts, 1980, pp 119–141 (40).)

stantia gelatinosa in suppression of cranial spread of dorsal root potentials. Hence, Lupa et al. (41) found that ipsilateral dorsal root potentials that are produced by stimulation of the L5 dorsal root and spread caudally attain only 47% of the amplitude observed at the L6 dorsal root by the time that they have passed six segments. Conversely, cranially spreading dorsal root potentials decreased to zero by the time they had passed six segments.

Antidromic activity may also help to dampen afferent noxious bombardment of the dorsal horns. Curtis et al. (42) have shown that *antidromic discharge* (i.e., nerve conduction that is opposite to the normal direction, e.g., from axon toward dendrites) in the dorsal horn results from the extracellular flow of current that is generated by the propagation of action potentials. These transient depolarizations of Type A alpha and beta afferent terminals synapsing on motoneurons act to lower the motoneuron threshold for conduction.

Further evidence that several phenomena may act to dampen or depress the afferent bombardment that may be associated with SF is found in a study by Calvin (43). They were able to demonstrate alteration in sensitivity to synaptic currents when repetitive firing occurs in neurons. According to these researchers, currents may be increased or decreased at the synapse by depression, facilitation, or posttetanic potentiation.

The dorsal funiculus and/or medial lemniscal pathway (viz. dorsal column system) is the primary pathway for proprioceptive impulses from joint and tendon receptors, once these impulses are in the spinal column. The dorsal column system is made up of large myelinated fast-conducting fibers that, according to McIntyre (44), carry muscle afferents (Type A beta, gamma and delta) to the cerebral cortex along with touch, phasic, vibratory, kinesthetic, and pressure sensations to the medulla, thalamus, and postcentral gyrus of the cerebral cortex.

It has been said that the primary pathway in the spine for nociceptive sensations is the lateral spinothalamic system (neospinothalamic tract). Although other tracts are functional in nociceptive discrimination (i.e., dorsal column system, spinocervicothalamic tract, paleospinothalamic tract, spinoreticular tract, and multisynaptic ascending propriospinal system), it has been said that the three discriminative ascending pain pathways are the neospinothalamic tract, the dorsal column system, and the spinocervicothalamic tract (40) (Figure 8.3). Of these, perhaps the best known is the lateral spinothalamic system. Although these fibers respond to Type A delta fiber stimulation as well as to Type C fiber stimulation, this tract may not be that important in the transfer

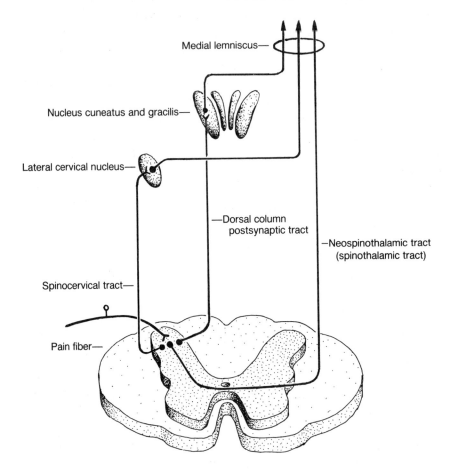

Figure 8.3. Three pathways for pain that are considered discriminative. The spinothalamic tract is considered the oldest known and perhaps the most direct pathway for nociception (pain). (Adapted from Haldeman S: Neurophysiology of spinal pain syndromes. In Haldeman S (ed): *Modern Developments in the Principles and Practice of Chiropractic.* New York, Appleton-Century-Crofts, 1980, pp 119–141 (40).)

of noxious stimuli, since few of these fibers actually even reach the thalamus; most terminate in the lower reticular formation (45). It has been demonstrated that Type A and C fiber stimulation affects both wide-dynamic-range and high-threshold spinothalamic tract cells. This system conveys, in addtion to pain, thermal, crude touch, pressure, tickle, itch, and sexual sensation to the reticular formation (45).

The important question with which we are faced is, Can segmental afferent bombardment of dorsal horn cells affect normal somatic and autonomic function? Coote (46) describes several pathways by which somatic sensations could affect normal sympathetic reflexes. In addition to synapsing directly in the tract of Lissauer, the small somatic and visceral afferents entering the dorsal horn may synapse in the substantia gelatinosa where synaptic contacts with Lissauer may occur for up to six segments; this feature involves somatosympathetic and viscerosympathetic reflexes (46). Those afferent impulses that reach laminae IV and V of the dorsal horn (which contributes to the dorsolateral system) may ascend via the ventral funiculus, anterolateral fasciculus, and dorsolateral funiculus. This pathway is especially important because it is the main ascending afferent pathway for sympathetic reflexes that have been mediated by medullary or supramedullary regions (46). The lamina V cells that receive inputs from both small somatic as well as small visceral afferent fibers (which are responsible for sympathetic reflexes) are perhaps the most interesting and revealing of all the neuronal pools (46). Gardner (29) delineated the role of the spinocervicothalamic tract in which input to the dorsolateral funiculus ascends to the lateral cervical nucleus where the impulses synapse before ending in the thalamic region.

Ample evidence suggests that somatic afferent input does indeed affect autonomic and somatic reflexes (47–51). Researchers have shown that supramaximal stimulation of forelimb muscle Type A delta fibers evoked small early responses in thoracic sympathetic nerves with latencies in the range of 92 to 157 msec (52). Corbett et al. (53) have shown that in humans (tetraplegic patients), muscle spasm can stimulate blood pressure and heart rate increases. Indeed, chronic spinal pain with its afferent bombardment may actually result in an increased arousal response, a decrease in the performance of difficult tasks which leads to pain (viz. a more sedentary lifestyle), and decreased evidence of muscle spasm (54). Hence, Collins et al. (54) determined that although chronic low back pain patients demonstrated significantly increased frontalis EMG and galvanic skin conductance (an auto-nomic response), they actually had similar or significantly less muscle spasm (paraspinal) than their matched controls.

There is much evidence that somatic afferent inputs remote from the level of sympathetic efferent activity may evoke specific sympathetic reflex responses. It is known that nonnoxious stimu-lation of the skin anywhere in the body, for example, produces sympathetic postganglionic activity at an increased level to cuta-neous vascular beds but at a decreased level to muscular vascular beds. Noxious stimulation of the skin, however, produces the opposite affects. Burgess and Perl (55) and Bessou and Perl (56) have demonstrated that both myelinated and unmyelinated fibers are necessary for relay of cutaneous noxious and innocuous ther-mal stimuli.

Coote (46) has established two important principles with regard to somatosympathetic reflexes: a) a spatial organization is seen in some somatosympathetic reflexes; and b) somatic afferent input can enter the cord at one segment, yet the relevant sympathetic preganglionic neurons may be located at an entirely different segmental level. Thus Beacham and Perl (57) were able to dem-onstrate that preganglionic units at one spinal level could be activated at a shorter latency by afferent input from an adjacent segment than by afferent input to the same segment. Numerous other experimental studies of this subject as well as a more complete discussion can be found in Chapter 11.

Korr Model of Spinal Fixation

From evaluation of years of research for the osteopathic profes-sion, Korr (11) developed a hypothesis regarding the propriocep-tive activity that could create muscle spasm and the fixation of segments seen in the osteopathic "lesion." Because the osteo-pathic "lesion" and the chiropractic "intervertebral subluxation" are analogous, the Korr model of spinal fixation (SF) is studied here. This area of the lesion is referred to as a SF.

Korr bases his model on the fact that spinal cord segments adjacent to the SF become *facilitated* (i.e., they have a lower threshold for firing). In this zone, which includes anterior and lateral horn cells as well as cells of ascending pain pathways, facilitation affects motor and autonomic function and nociception.

These neurons become hyperresponsive to input from the brain and the body. According to Korr, both afferents from the musculoskeletal tissues adjacent to the SF and visceral afferents may be involved in this facilitation.

Korr discounts the role of joint receptors in his hypothesis, stating that little evidence suggests that joint receptors can influence motor activity. Instead, he focuses on the muscle spindle as the coordinator that may increase or decrease muscle contraction according to the direction of motion of the joint. This reflex muscle contraction can then produce joint motion by its action or prevent joint motion in an area of SF.

The mechanism Korr uses to explain such a phenomenon involves the fusimotor background discharge that is seen during Type A alpha motoneuron activity. Korr explains that the CNS adjusts the slack in the muscle spindle that occurs during extrafusal contraction by adjusting the level of background activity in the fusimotor system. Not only is the slack in the spindle taken up by increased gamma motor activity, but the CNS turns the level of background activity up or down according to the needs of the muscle. For example, the athlete who wishes to swing a bat or a hockey stick in a wide arc must have a method of "pre-setting" the gamma activity in his muscles so that large changes in muscle length may be swiftly and smoothly accomplished. In this example, the CNS would turn down the level of background activity in the fusimotor system of the involved muscles so that as the skeletal muscles contract gradually, there will be only a gradual simultaneous contraction of the intrafusal fibers. On the other hand, the tennis player who plays the net must have this background activity increased in order to return the ball with a minimum of muscle motion. In this way, the CNS can set and reset spindle sensitivity through the fusimotor system. Korr calls this a type of automatic "gain" which controls the length-regulating mechanism for each skeletal muscle.

Sometimes, cerebral influences may set the spindle sensitivity at the wrong level for correct muscular activity. Tension and stressful situations may result in the "gain" being set too high; muscles may be tense and resistant to change in length and, according to the Korr hypothesis, the person is said to be "jumpy" or "irritable."

With the idea of "gain" kept in mind, it is easy to visualize the
main points of the Korr hypothesis (Figure 8.4):

1. The CNS orders skeletal muscle contraction (which carries
   with it background low "gain" gamma motoneuron activity).

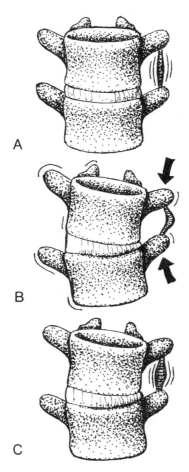

Figure 8.4.   Schema of the Korr (11) model of SF. *A.* CNS orders skeletal muscle
contraction. *B.* At the same time, vertebral attachments are approximated by
external forces, etc. (this has the effect of silencing annulospiral receptor
activity). *C.* CNS turns up the gammomotoneuron "gain," thereby increasing the
intensity of the contraction. Due to this contraction, the vertebral attachments
cannot return to their normal position; gravity and postural reflexes further
stretch the muscle, which causes continued resistance and high "gain" or "spasm"
activity.

2. At the same time, vertebral attachments are suddenly approximated (by external forces or by the unexpected withdrawal of a load or force that is opposing strong isometric extrafusal contraction), which results in slackening of the muscle spindles quickly and, thereby, silencing of the annulospiral activity.

3. Without an annulospiral report, the CNS assumes that the gamma motor "gain" is not set high enough for the primary receptor endings to transmit the impulses for the contraction. The CNS then turns up the "gain" to compensate for this discrepancy. Increasing the gamma motor activity likewise results in increased fusimotor activity, and the muscle is contracted further.

4. As the body recoils from the forced motion and the vertebral attachments attempt to return to their normal position, they find that they are now opposed in this by the now resistant muscle. The joint surfaces are approximated, and increased frictional resistance prevents normal motion.

5. Gravity and postural reflexes tend to stretch the muscle to resting length, and the joint receptors continue to report their true position. The high "gain" activity, however, causes the muscle to resist, and the muscle is in a state of "spasm."

According to the hypothesis, the relative lengths of the intrafusal and extrafusal fibers have been increased by centrally ordered fusimotor activity in the area of the SF. Therefore, reduction of gamma motor discharge will be the central aim in producing increased mobility and thereby correction through chiropractic adjustments. Korr proposed two mechanisms whereby manipulation would successfully turn down the "gain" and thereby relax the muscle spasm. First, stretch of the intrafusal fibers by forcefully stretching the muscle against its spindle-maintained resistance would produce a barrage of afferent impulses of sufficient intensity so as to signal the CNS to reduce the gamma motoneuron discharge. Second, the Golgi tendon organs would be stimulated by forced stretch of the skeletal muscle causing gamma as well as alpha motoneuron inhibition. Korr predicts that both the slow-range-of-motion, long-lever type of manipulation and the rapid, high-velocity, short-lever type of chiropractic adjustment would be successful in stretching the muscles against their resistance.

Discussion

It is becoming increasingly evident that the CNS, rather than responding to individual fibers, responds to patterns of firing. This idea is consistent with the idea of neuronal pools that sort out the input and disregard that which is unessential. Indeed, Guyton (28) estimated that more than 99% of all the information that the brain receives is discarded as unimportant. The various phenomena described in this chapter are functional in the processing of unessential information, but the sympathetic reflexes and other somatic reflexes must certainly be affected to some degree by the somatic afferent bombardment seen in an area of spinal fixation (14–19, 21, 26, 27). This must be so in order to explain the findings of many independent experimental studies (46–53, 55–57) (see Chapter 11). Korr (11) has shown us a model of what might happen to initiate and maintain a SF. His high-gain gamma motoneuron hypothesis is more than reasonable from an analytic point of view. Lewit (23), however, in a convincing although small study has presented data that contradicts the Korr model. Lewit examined the cervical spine of patients who were prepared for operation. These individuals were reexamined under general anesthesia which included myorelaxants and intubation with artificial respiration. Movement restriction was even more recognizable during narcosis in 10 patients, as they were totally relaxed. Lewit took this as conclusive proof that the movement restriction was not in the muscle. The fact that proprioceptive information contributes more to the perception of joint displacements and faster antagonist reaction in muscle than does cutaneous input, further suggests that joint fixation may not be necessarily dependent on muscle spasm (58).

The data indicate that although it is probably not possible at this time to produce a foolproof model of spinal fixation, such a phenomenon does exist and has been documented clinically as well as experimentally. It has been suggested that this hypothesis, if proven, may be the most reasonable justification for the use of chiropractic adjustments in disorders other than pain syndromes (10, 11). Possibly this conclusion has been reached because the nerve root compression hypothesis and the cord compression and vertebrobasilar arterial insufficiency (VBAI) hypotheses could not reasonably apply to most cases of functional or pathological diseases when somatoautonomic reflexes are involved (see Chapters 6, 7, and 9). In contrast, the SF has been shown to affect sympathetic reflexes as well as somatic transmission (14-19, 21, 26, 27, 46-53, 55-57).

It should be understood that the organization of the CNS into neuronal pools that weigh groups of patterns, as well as the phenomena of descending inhibition, antidromic discharge, etc., may influence the outcome or pathogenesis of the SF. (28, 37, 42-45). Because of the complex nature of the CNS involvement, it is very difficult to predict the effect of any particular SF on autonomic or other function (20, 28, 37-45, 54, 58, 59).

Summary

The spinal fixation (SF) as a clinical phenomenon has been the subject of clinical and experimental research (2-5, 10-19, 21-27, 44). The afferent somatic bombardment of dorsal horn cells, which is theoretically produced by the SF, may well affect various somatosomatic and somatoautonomic reflexes (10-13, 18, 19, 21-27, 46-53, 55-57). The Korr (11) hypothesis of SF has been presented as a model of the phenomenon, although it is understood that this model may not be entirely correct (23). It is concluded that the SF is likely to create some degree of interruption of normal neural transmission within the CNS, although the phenomena of neuronal pools, descending inhibition, antidromic discharge, etc., make it difficult at best to predict the effect of any given SF on CNS function (28, 37, 42-45).

References

1. Schmorl G, Junghanns H: *The Human Spine in Health and Disease,* ed. 2. New York, Grune & Stratton, 1971, pp 221-222.
2. Janse JH, Wells BF: *Chiropractic Principles and Technic.* Chicago, National College of Chiropractic, 1947.
3. Wright HM: *Perspectives in Osteopathic Medicine.* Kirksville, MO, Kirksville College of Osteopathic Medicine, 1976.
4. Giles LGF: Spinal fixations and viscera. *J Clin Chiropractic Arch* 3:144-165, 1973.
5. Inman OB: *Basic Chiropractic Procedural Manual.* Des Moines, American Chiropractic Association, 1973.
6. Verner JR: *The Science and Logic of Chiropractic.* Brooklyn, Cerasoli, 1941.
7. Korr IM: Sustained sympathicotonia as a factor in disease. In Korr IM (ed): *The Neurobiologic Mechanisms in Manipulative Therapy.* New York, Plenum, 1978, pp 229-268.
8. Homewood AE: *The Neurodynamics of the Vertebral Subluxation.* St. Petersburg, Valkyrie Press, 1979, p 163.

9. Hviid H: A consideration of contemporary chiropractic theory. *J Natl Chiropractic Assoc* 25:17-18, 1955.
10. Haldeman S: The clinical basis for discussion of mechanisms of manipulative therapy. In Korr IM (ed): *The Neurobiologic Mechanisms in Manipulative Therapy*. New York, Plenum, 1978, pp 53-75.
11. Korr IM: Proprioceptors and the behavior of lesioned segments. In Stark EH (ed): *Osteopathic Medicine*. Acton, MA, Publication Sciences Group, 1975, pp 183-199.
12. Haldeman S: Spinal and paraspinal receptors. *J Can Chiropractic Assoc* 17:28-32, 1972.
13. Haldeman S: The neurophysiological mechanisms of pain. *ACA J Chiropractic* 10:53-64, 1976.
14. Northup GW: History of the development of osteopathic concepts; osteopathic terminology. In Goldstein M (ed): *The Research Status of Spinal Manipulative Therapy*. Washington, DC, Government Printing Office, 1975, pp 43-52.
15. Gillet H, Liekens M: Fixation analysis-movement palpation. In Kfoury P (ed): *Catalog of Chiropractic Techniques*. St. Louis, Logan College of Chiropractic, 1977, pp 101-102.
16. Stoner F: *The Eclectic Approach to Chiropractic*. Las Vegas, FLS Publications, 1975.
17. Nimmo RL: Receptor-tonus method. In Kfoury P (ed): *Catalog of Chiropractic Techniques*. St. Louis, Logan College of Chiropractic, 1977, pp 63-64.
18. Denslow JS, Hassett CC: The central excitatory state associated with postural abnormalities. *J Neurophysiol* 5:393-402, 1942.
19. Denslow JS: An analysis of the variability of spinal reflex thresholds. *J Neurophysiol* 7:207-215, 1944.
20. Denslow JS, Korr IM, Krems AD: Quantitative studies of chronic facilitation in human motoneuron pools. *Am J Physiol* 150:229-238, 1947.
21. Janda V: Muscles, central nervous system motor regulation and back problems. In Korr IM (ed): *The Neurobiologic Mechanisms in Manipulative Therapy*. New York, Plenum, 1978, pp 27-41.
22. Janda V: Postural and phasic muscles in the pathogenesis of low back pain. In: *Proceedings of the Eleventh Congress, International Society for Rehabilitation of the Disabled*. Dublin, International Society for Rehabilitation of the Disabled, 1969, pp 553-554.
23. Lewit K: The contribution of clinical observation to neurobiological mechanisms in manipulative therapy. In Korr IM (ed): *The Neurobiologic Mechanisms in Manipulative Therapy*. New York, Plenum, 1978, pp 43-52.
24. Greenman PE: Manipulative therapy in relation to total health care. In Korr IM (ed): *The Neurobiologic Mechanisms in Manipulative Therapy*. New York, Plenum, 1978, pp 43-52.
25. Drum D: The vertebral motor unit and intervertebral foramen. In Goldstein M (ed): *The Research Status of Spinal Manipulative Therapy*. Washington, DC, Government Printing Office, 1975, pp 63-75.
26. England R, Deibert P: Electromyographic studies, Part 1: Consideration in the evaluation of osteopathic therapy. *J Am Osteopath Assoc* 72:162-169, 1972.
27. Grice A: Muscle tonus changes following manipulation. *J Can Chiropractic Assoc* 19:29-31, 1974.
28. Guyton A: *Basic Human Physiology*. Philadelphia, Saunders, 1971.
29. Gardner E: Pathways to the cerebral cortex for nerve impulses from joints. *Acta Anat [Suppl]* 56:203-216, 1969.
30. Warwick R, Williams P (eds): *Gray's Anatomy*, ed 35. Philadelphia, Saunders, 1973, pp 784 and 786.
31. Chusid JG: *Correlative Neuroanatomy and Functional Neurology*. Los Altos, CA, Lange, 1973.

32. Willer JC, Boureau F, Albe-Fessard D: Role of large diameter cutaneous afferents in transmission of nociceptive messages: electrophysiological study in man. *Brain Res* 152:358–364, 1978.

33. LaMotte RH, Campbell J: Comparison of responses of warm and nociceptive C-fiber afferents in monkey with human judgments of thermal pain. *J Neurophysiol* 41:509–528, 1978.

34. Novikoff AB, Holtzman E: *Cells and Organelles.* New York, Holt, Rinehart & Winston, 1976.

35. Villee CA, Walker WF, Barnes RD: *General Zoology,* ed 5. Philadelphia, Saunders, 1978, pp 372–374.

36. Burke D, Hagbarth K-E, Lofstedt L: Muscle spindle activity in man during shortening and lengthening contraction. *J Physiol* 277:131–142, 1978.

37. Holloway JA, Keyser GF, Wright LE, Trouth CO: Supraspinal inhibition of dorsal horn cell activity and location of descending pathways in the chicken (*Gallus domesticus*). *Brain Res* 145:380–384, 1978.

38. Carstens E, Klumpp D, Zimmermann M: Differential inhibitory effects on medial and lateral midbrain stimulation on spinal neuronal discharges to noxious skin heating in the cat. *J Neurophysiol* 43:332–342, 1980.

39. Carstens E, Bihl H, Irvine DRF, Zimmerman M: Descending inhibition from medial and lateral midbrain of spinal dorsal horn neuronal responses to noxious and nonnoxious cutaneous stimuli in the cat. *J Neurophysiol* 45:1029–1042, 1981.

40. Haldeman S: Neurophysiology of spinal pain syndromes. In Haldeman S (ed): *Modern Developments in the Principles and Practice of Chiropractic.* New York, Appleton-Century-Crofts, 1980, pp 119–141.

41. Lupa K, Wojcik G, Ozog M, Niechaj A: Spread of the dorsal root potentials in lower lumbar, sacral and upper caudal spinal cord. *Eur J Physiol* 381:201–207, 1979.

42. Curtis DR, Lodge D, Headley PM: Electrical interaction between motoneurons and afferent terminals in cat spinal cord. *J Neurophysiol* 42:635–641, 1979.

43. Calvin WH: Setting the pace and pattern of discharge: Do CNS neurons vary their sensitivity to external inputs via their repetitive firing processes? *Fed Proc* 37:2165–2170, 1978.

44. McIntyre A: Central projections of impulses from receptors activated by muscle stretch. *Symposium on Muscle Receptors.* Hong Kong, Hong Kong University Press, 1962.

45. Chung JM, Kenshalo DR, Gerhart KD, Willis WD: Excitation of primate spinothalamic neurons by cutaneous C-fiber volleys. *J Neurophysiol* 42:1354–1369, 1979.

46. Coote JH: Somatic sources of afferent input as factors in aberrant autonomic, sensory and motor function. In Korr IM (ed): *The Neurobiologic Mechanisms in Manipulative Therapy.* New York, Plenum, 1978, pp 91–127.

47. Sato A, Schmidt RF: Somatosympathetic reflexes: afferent fibers, central pathways, discharge characteristics. *Physiol Rev* 53:916–947, 1973.

48. Sato A: The somatosympathetic reflexes: their physiological and clinical significance. In Goldstein M (ed): *The Research Status of Spinal Manipulative Therapy.* Washington, DC, Government Printing Office, 1975, pp 163–172.

49. King DW, Green JB: Short latency somatosensory potentials in humans. *Electroencephalogr Clin Neurophysiol* 46:702–708, 1979.

50. Goldberg LJ, Yoshio N: Production of primary afferent depolarization in group Ia fibers from the masseter muscle by stimulation of trigeminal cutaneous afferents. *Brain Res* 134:561–567, 1977.

51. Haldeman S: Interactions between the somatic and visceral nervous systems. *ACA J Chiropractic* 5:57–64, 1971.

52. Whitwam JG, Kidd C, Fussey IV: Responses in sympathetic nerves of the dog evoked by stimulation of somatic nerves. *Brain Res* 165:219–233, 1979.

53. Corbett JL, et al: Cardiovascular changes associated with skeletal muscle spasm in tetraplegic man. *J Physiol* 215:381–393, 1971.

54. Collins G, Cohen MJ, Naliboff BD, Schandler SL: Comparative analysis of paraspinal and frontalis EMG, heart rate and skin conductance in chronic low back pain patients and normals to various postures and stress. *Scand J Rehabil Med* 14:39–46, 1982.

55. Burgess PR, Perl ER: Myelinated afferent fibers responding specifically to noxious stimulation of the skin. *J Physiol* 190:541–562, 1967.

56. Bessou P, Perl ER: Response of cutaneous sensory units with unmyelinated fibers to noxious stimuli. *J Neurophysiol* 32:1025–1043, 1969.

57. Beacham WS, Perl ER: Background and reflex discharge of sympathetic preganglionic neurones in the spinal cat. *J Physiol* 172:400–416, 1964.

58. Bawa P, McKenzie DC: Contribution of joint and cutaneous afferents to longer-latency reflexes in man. *Brain Res* 211:185–189, 1981.

59. Coote JH: Central organization of somatosympathetic reflexes. In Haldeman S (ed): *Modern Developments in the Principles and Practice of Chiropractic.* New York, Appleton-Century-Crofts, 1980, pp 107–118.

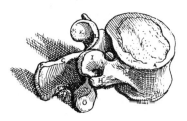

Chapter 9

Hypothesis of Vertebrobasilar Arterial Insufficiency

*M*any patients apparently seek and obtain relief from such conditions as migraine, dizziness, and other complaints localized to the cranial region by utilizing chiropractic care, but the mechanism for such relief is disputed (1–4). Palmer (4) stated that by racking the bones of the spine into their proper alignment, a man's hearing was restored. He believed that nerves compressed by the intervertebral foramen at their root had resulted in the hearing loss. Christensen (5) cited work by medical specialists in Denmark, including one series of seven patients with hearing deficit who were successfully treated by cervical manipulation. Haldeman (6) has performed an extensive review of the literature concerning the influence of the autonomic nervous system (ANS) on cerebral blood flow. He came to the conclusion that the ANS appears to affect cerebral blood flow to some degree. ANS influence, however, would not be severe enough to seriously compromise the nutrient supply to nervous system tissue. Haldeman has, therefore, indicated that there is no proof that chiropractic adjustment can affect the innervation to the blood vessels of the cranium in a magnitude that would give rise to symptoms there. There is, however, another mechanism whereby adjustment of the cervical vertebrae directly affects a considerable portion of cerebral blood flow.

Various medical researchers have determined that injury to the cervical spine, congenital anomalies, spondylosis (atherosclerosis, arteriosclerosis of vertebral arteries), and subluxation of the cervical vertebrae may result in deflection or compression of the vertebral arteries (7–20). In some rare cases, embolism within the higher cerebral vessels may result in stroke, other neurologic deficit(s), and death (21–32). More recently, chiropractors have noticed that this vertebrobasilar arterial insufficiency syndrome may be caused by cervical disrelationships (33–35). The hypothesis that cervical intervertebral subluxations may cause deflection or compression of the vertebral arteries, which thereby gives rise to altered cerebral blood supply, is termed the hypothesis of vertebrobasilar arterial insufficiency (VBAI). Medical doctors have suggested that manipulation may initiate the syndrome, and chiropractic researchers agree that there is strong evidence confirming that the presence of the syndrome is a contraindication for adjustment or manipulation (21–32, 36). It is suggested by this author that when subluxations are the etiology of this syndrome, chiropractic adjustments may be useful in correction of it. It is acknowledged, however, that under certain conditions adjustment is contraindicated. It is suggested that this may be the mechanism whereby chiropractic adjustment corrects symptoms referable to the cranium.

Characteristics of VBAI

Typically, an osteophyte, subluxation, or fracture/dislocation of a cervical vertebra (usually atlantoaxial) initiates a peculiar complex of symptoms by compressing or deflecting a vertebral artery as it passes through the involved foramen transversarium (7–12) (Figure 9.1). Congenital bony anomalies and anomalies in the origin of the vertebral artery have also been associated with this syndrome (15, 20). The vertebral arteries comprise a very considerable portion of the blood supply to the cranium (17–18). Perhaps more importantly, these vessels comprise the major blood supply to the brain stem (9). Symptoms have been previously described as the Barré-Lieau syndrome and include headache, nausea, vomiting, nystagmus, and suboccipital tenderness (12). A more complete picture includes dizziness and "drop attacks" (instantaneous and temporary quadriplegia on rotation and extension of the neck) (9, 13–16). Arteriosclerotic involvement may result in hemorrhage of the tunica media and cause a dissecting

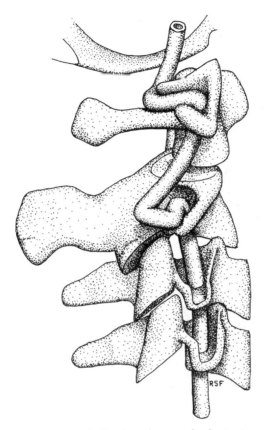

Figure 9.1. In the upper cervical spine, the vertebral arteries are most susceptible to deflection and obstruction by subluxation (including, especially, atlas
laterality as well as articular process slippage to below the level of the transverse
process), osteophytic spurring, increased tortuosity from lower cervical degenerative joint disease, and even cervical spine manipulation itself.

aneurysm, effectively shutting off the lumen of the vertebral artery
(11, 16). Whether atheromatous changes develop in compressed
vessels following chronic subluxation, etc. (12, 16), or they develop incidentally, further trauma may induce subintimal hemorrhage sufficient to complete the occlusion (11).

Role of Subluxation in Etiology of VBAI

Various researchers have documented the role of subluxation
in causing VBAI. Jackson associates lateral atlas subluxation with

constriction of the vertebral arteries as they course through the transverse foramina (7):

> Relaxation or stretching of the guy ligaments may allow lateral sub luxation of the head of the atlas on the axis and excessive rotation of the axis in its relationship to the head of the atlas, and may be responsible for irritation of the vertebral arteries as they wind around the atlanto-axial joints and the superior facets of the atlas.

Jackson believed that constriction of these vessels most often occurs in the upper cervical (atlas, axis, third cervical) spine where they are most susceptible to trauma (whiplash, sporting injuries, etc.). She recognized that such constriction produces vascular insufficiency to the brain with subsequent dysfunction. Furthermore, she stated that the sympathetic nerve supply to these vessels, following trauma, may initiate a persistent vasoconstriction that may develop into permanent narrowing and complete constriction. Further vascular insufficiency of the spinal cord may result if vasoconstriction or narrowing of the anterior and posterior spinal arteries (cranial branches of the vertebral arteries) occurs in addition to vertebral artery involvement.

Kovacs (8) has determined from clinical and cadaver studies that subluxation in the cervical spine is possibly a common factor in the etiology of VBAI. He has associated the syndrome with chronic and other forms of headaches (8):

> We believe that headache radiating from the top of the skull and the nuchal region[,] as well as the upper cervical sympathetic syndrome described by Barré-Lieau, is more frequently produced by pressure exerted on the vertebral artery and nerve by the superior articular process than by other conditions.

Kovacs found slippage of the articular process to below the level of the transverse process in 22 of 40 chronic headache sufferers. For 20 of these 22, anteflexion-traction was found radiographically to correct the subluxation and subjectively to relieve the headache. Kovacs studied 54 postmortem cases. He demonstrated chronic subluxations by radiography and, at postmortem examination, found bony excavation within the transverse foramina, where the pulsating vertebral arteries had actually etched into the bones. The studies of Kovacs thus document dramatically the role of subluxation in causing headaches.

Schneider and Schemm (9) have recognized the role of atlas-axis and atlas-occiput dislocation in producing the vertebral artery compression syndrome. They believed that either the aforementioned dislocations or direct contusion of the spinal cord results in spinal cord and neurologic involvement. They explained that when the vertebral arteries become compressed within the transverse foramen of a dislocated or fractured atlas, the blood supply to the circle of Willis (circulus arteriosus cerebri) and hence the anterior spinal artery is then inhibited. A resultant hypoxia of the spinal cord then ensues with increased motor activity to the lower extremities (relative to the upper extremities) and varied sensory findings. Paralysis lasting from minutes to days was noted by these authors.

Seletz (10) described the brief posterior subluxation that occurs in whiplash cases. He believed that symptoms of vertigo, ataxia, diplopia, severe attacks of migraine headache, hemicrania with nausea and vomiting, and transient disturbance of speech and swallowing were due to compromised circulation of the vertebral arteries following neck sprain or whiplash.

Gurdjian et al. (11) described five cases of carotid and vertebral artery involvement following various types of accidents. Fracture/dislocation of cervical vertebrae was found to be associated with vertebral artery involvement. In one case of vertebral artery compression, there were no signs of brain stem or cerebellar involvement. The authors believed that in this case the artery being compressed was already congenitally small; further occlusion of it, therefore, did not sufficiently inhibit blood flow to the circle of Willis.

Hadley (12) has implicated grossly hyperplastic arthrotic posterior vertebral joints as a cause of vertebral artery compression. Such subluxations are, according to Kovacs (8), of a chronic and irreparable nature.

Other Etiologies of VBAI

Husni et al. (13) found basilar artery insufficiency in 20 patients reporting dizziness. The dizziness was traced to vertebral artery occlusion at the fifth and sixth cerebral vertebrae. Only patients in whom lateral rotation of the neck resulted in vertebral artery occlusion were included in this study. In 18 of the patients the vertebral artery on one side was congenitally smaller than that on the other side; in every patient in whom unilateral blockage of the vessel produced symptoms, it was the larger artery that was blocked. The frequency of disparity between vertebral artery diameters in the same person is quite high. Stein et al. (14) found that in 45 of 130 postmortem examinations the right vertebral artery was smaller than the left. Only in 59 examinations were the arteries in the same cadaver of equal diameter. Husni et al. found that during surgery, tension on certain interdigitations of tendons resulted in compression of the involved vertebral artery. These were the tendinous slips of origin of the longus colli and scalenus medius muscles. By sectioning the tendons and interposing a pedicle to prevent regrowth, these surgeons attained dramatic symptomatic and objective improvement in nearly all their patients. These were patients who had suffered dizziness, vertigo, headaches, and loss of consciousness as well as gait and visual disturbance, nausea, numbness, and scalenus anticus before the operations. The authors concluded that in patients who suffered VBAI syndrome on simple rotation and extension of the neck, the cause is a mechanical obstruction by tendons and can be corrected with surgery.

Anderson et al. (15), however, reported on a patient in whom simple rotation of the neck to the right side and upward (no dislocations or osteophytes observable) resulted in marked occlusion of the left vertebral artery. In this patient, the right vertebral artery was hypoplastic, and the left vessel was of an anomalous origin (from the aortic arch medially to the origin of the subclavian artery). This 37-year-old man suffered headaches, vertigo, and nystagmus which were markedly aggravated by the previously described neck movement.

In a comprehensive study of the subject, Sheehan et al. (16) concluded that cervical spondylosis was the primary etiology of vertebrobasilar arterial compression syndrome. They found that a common form of the syndrome occurs when spondylosis (with osteophytic encroachment of the vertebral artery) and cerebrovascular atherosclerosis are combined. They also found vertebral artery occlusion in 26 of 46 patients with recurrent cerebrovascular symptoms and/or cervical spondylosis. Rotation of the neck resulted in further narrowing or complete occlusion of the vessel on the same side on which the osteophyte was compressing the artery. In addition to osteophytes, it was found angiographically that atheromatous plaques (3 patients) and arteriosclerotic tortuosity (10 patients) were other factors associated with this syndrome. A significantly greater occurrence of spondylotic vertebral artery compression was found in men than in women. A special complaint of some patients was sudden, transient quadriparesis with subsequent falling to the ground (no loss of consciousness). This "drop attack" was believed to be pathognomonic for the syndrome. Interestingly, these authors were in accord with Kovacs (6) who found signs of nerve root and cord compression in some patients with subluxation as well as VBAI.

Tatlow and Bammer (17) have cited three cases in which rotation of the neck resulted in neurologic signs and symptoms referable to VBAI. In this early study, it was demonstrated on postmortem examination that rotation and extension of the neck on the involved side, when combined with vascular abnormalities or the presence of osteophytes, resulted in occlusion of the vertebral artery. Anticoagulant therapy was successful in clinical cases when trauma in the presence of arteriosclerosis had resulted in thrombus formation higher up in the cerebral arteries. This was the mechanism which was hypothesized to explain certain cases of stroke and death following cervical manipulation.

Other authors (14, 18, 19) have documented that one of the most common causes of VBAI syndrome is atheromatous plaques.

Barton and Margolis (20) documented two other cases of VBAI syndrome caused by rotational obstruction at the atlantoaxial joint. These researchers found that rotational obstruction only initiates this syndrome when the contralateral vertebral artery is already compromised (congenitally).

Contraindication for Chiropractic Adjustment

It has been acknowledged by medical (21–30) and chiropractic (31, 32, 36) researchers that in the presence of certain predisposing factors, cervical manipulation may result in thrombus formation, ischemia, stroke, and death. This apparently is a rare complication of cervical spine manipulation, having been reported approximately 11 times in the last four decades (according to rough estimates, based on 50 million manipulations yearly over the past 40 years, the odds of this complication occurring are 1 death/181 million adjustments (21–26, 31, 37) Even if the number of unreported cases is quadruple the number of reported cases, this mechanism is rare. It has been stated, however, that up to 45 cases of vertebrobasilar infarction have resulted from chiropractic manipulation alone, 34 of which resulted in moderate to serious sequelae not including death (27, 31). As there have been complications reported from medical, physical therapist, and osteopathic manipulations as well, awareness and identification of this mechanism is important.

According to the medical literature, the typical case involves a patient who receives a standard rotary cervical adjustment or manipulation. Predisposing factors that have been reported include:

1. Unilateral vertebral artery obstruction by congenital or developmental factors. When the contralateral artery is then diminished by the rotary and extension movements found in cervical spine manipulation, both arteries then become obstructed. Such factors include arteriosclerosis, vascular anomaly, and unilateral vertebral artery occlusion.
2. Degenerative joint disease, even in the lower cervical spine, can result in a loss of disc height which shortens the cervical spine and allows the vertebral arteries to become more tortuous. This condition may effectively reduce the lumen of these vessels, which predisposes them to further occlusion by cervical spine manipulation.
3. Osteophytic outgrowths, especially from the zygapophyses, can obstruct the course of the vertebral arteries. In this case, cervical spine manipulation on the side of the osteophytic outgrowths reduces the flow through the artery on the same side.

Manipulation of a patient who has one or more of these predisposing factors may then result in thrombus formation, ischemia, and stroke, especially in the presence of vascular disease (21–30, 32). Giles (36) has taken the position that a differential diagnosis of VBAI syndrome is a contraindication to regular chiropractic adjustment. He believed that the Cyriax method of careful manipulation during strong traction is a better form of treatment for these predisposed individuals. Giles stated that bed rest, limitation of neck movement and, possibly, intervention with anticoagulants or surgical procedures (depending on the severity of the condition) are the treatments of choice for patients with VBAI syndrome. Therefore, he basically is in accord with Sheehan et al. (16) on the course of treatment.

A recent case of cerebrovascular infarction in a 16-year-old boy who fell asleep with his head rotated to the left and extended is noteworthy (29). In this patient with congenitally anomalous vertebral artery distribution, the entire blood supply to the left occipital cortex was derived from the right vertebral artery. That normal physiologic head movements can result in cerebrovascular infarction in predisposed individuals underscores the necessity of identification of predisposed individuals prior to introduction of chiropractic manipulative therapy.

Clinical Considerations

Researchers have stated that VBAI is a relatively common syndrome (7–13). From their point of view, it is considered an etiology of a bizarre group of symptoms including dizziness; vertigo; nystagmus; ataxia; "drop attacks" considered pathognomonic of the syndrome; chronic, acute, and migraine headache; acute quadraparesis; hemicrania; nausea; vomiting; and disturbances of speech, swallowing and, possibly, balance. Although some investigators (7–12) have directly associated this syndrome with cervical subluxation, all recognize a host of other etiologies including osteophytes, abnormal presence of only one vertebral artery or one congenitally stenotic vessel, abnormal tortuosity of one or both vertebral arteries (as occurs in arteriosclerosis), other vascular disease such as atherosclerosis, and congenital bony anomalies and anomalies in origin of the vessels (7–20). The appearance of any combination of the aforementioned symptoms or clinical signs, especially when these were initiated or made severe by hyperextension and rotation of the neck, indicated the possible presence of the VBAI syndrome (7–17). The differential diagnosis includes Ménière's disease, certain brain tumors, and other disease and functional states causing dizziness or vertigo (36). A test useful in determining the presence of this syndrome has been described (36). In this test, the patient stands with eyes closed and arms stretched forward (horizontally) and is asked to rotate the head fully to one side and hold that position for 1 minute. This is repeated for the other side. Sway of the outstretched arms suggests cerebral ischemia caused by cervical rotation (36). A tentative diagnosis of VBAI suggests careful chiropractic management, and in the presence of atherosclerotic or arteriosclerotic phenomena, standard adjustment may be contraindicated (19–32, 36).

Discussion

Conflicting ideas are prevalent among the researchers involved in the study of this syndrome. Some investigators are critical of the chiropractic profession because cases of stroke and death following chiropractic adjustment of the neck have been reported (21–30). These cases are extremely rare, however (under a dozen reported incidences in four decades). In fact, other researchers have associated this syndrome with subluxations of cervical vertebrae (7–12). This implies that subluxation may be associated with a wide variety of symptoms referable to the cranium. The hypothesis of VBAI becomes important in light of the position held by Haldeman (6) and other researchers who have shown that sympathetic tone plays a minor role in cerebral blood flow and, hence, that mechanisms based on a neurovascular connection are questionable (38). Since chiropractors make their prime objective the correction of subluxations, it appears probable that they may be playing a role in correcting this condition. At any rate, there appears to be conclusive evidence to suggest that cervical intervertebral subluxations may indeed cause VBAI, especially in the presence of spondylosis (7–20). In this regard, we may assume that the hypothesis of VBAI is worthy of study as a mechanism that may explain the role of chiropractic in correcting certain cases of migraine as well as numerous other conditions of a cervicocranial origin.

Summary

The vertebrobasilar arterial insufficiency (VBAI) syndrome results from a variety of conditions including subluxation (7–20). The rotation and extension movements of the neck may initiate or aggravate the syndrome and result in "drop attacks" and symptoms including, typically, dizziness (13–16). Chiropractic adjustments or other manipulations appear to initiate the syndrome in some rare cases (21–30). A test is described to identify the syndrome (in addition to neck movements of rotation and extension) (36). It is hypothesized that chiropractors may be inadvertently correcting this condition in many individuals, by correcting subluxations.

References

1. Watkins RJ: The neurological first aid kit. *Chiropractic Econ* May/June 1970.
2. Janse J: History of the development of chiropractic concepts; chiropractic terminology. In Goldstein M (ed): *The Research Status of Spinal Manipulative Therapy.* Washington, DC, Government Printing Office, 1975, pp 25–42.
3. Parker GB, Tupling H, Pryor DS: Proceedings of the Australian Association of Manipulative Medicine. *Aust NZ J Med* 8:589, 1978.
4. Palmer DD: *The Science, Art and Philosophy of Chiropractic.* Portland, OR, Portland Printing House, 1910, p 18.
5. Christensen F: An updated study of chiropractic in Danish medicine. *Eur J Chiropractic* 31:86–99, 1983.
6. Haldeman S: The influence of the autonomic nervous system on cerebral blood flow. *J Can Chiropractic Assoc* 19:6–12, and 14, 1974.
7. Jackson R: *The Cervical Syndrome.* Springfield, IL, Charles C Thomas, 1978.
8. Kovacs A: Subluxation and deformation of the cervical apophyseal joints. *Acta Radiol* 43:1–15, 1955.
9. Schneider RC, Schemm GW: Vertebral artery insufficiency in acute and chronic spinal trauma. *J Neurosurg* 18:348–360, 1961.
10. Seletz E: Whiplash injuries—neurophysiological basis for pain and methods used for rehabilitation. *JAMA* 168:1750–1755, 1958.
11. Gurdjian EX, Hardy WG, Lindner DW, Thomas LM: Closed cervical cranial trauma associated with involvement of carotid and vertebral arteries. *J Neurosurg* 20:418–427, 1963.
12. Hadley LA: *Anatomico-Roentgenographic Studies of the Spine.* Springfield, IL, Charles C Thomas, 1964, pp 158–171.
13. Husni EA, Bell HS, Storer J: Mechanical occlusion of the vertebral artery. *JAMA* 196:475–478, 1966.
14. Stein BM, McCormick WF, Rodriguez JN, Taveras JM: Postmortem angiography of cerebral vascular system. *Arch Neurol* 7:545–559, 1962.
15. Anderson R, Carleson R, Nylen O: Vertebral artery insufficiency and rotational obstruction. *Acta Med Scand* 188:475–477, 1970.
16. Sheehan S, Bauer RB, Meyer JS: Vertebral artery compression in cervical spondylosis. *Neurology (Minneap)* 10:968–986, 1960.
17. Tatlow WFT, Bammer HG: Syndrome of vertebral artery compression. *Neurology (Minneap)* 7:331–340, 1957.
18. Bauer RB, Sheehan S, Meyer JS: Arteriographic study of cerebrovascular disease. *Arch Neurol* 4:119–131, 1961.
19. Faris AA, Poser CM, Wilmore DW, Agnew CH: Radiological visualization of neck vessels in healthy men. Neurology *(Minneap)* 13:386–396, 1963.
20. Barton JW, Margolis JW: Rotational obstruction of the vertebral artery at the atlantoaxial joint. *Neuroradiology* 9:117–120, 1975.
21. Green D, Joynt RJ: Vascular accidents to the brain stem associated with neck manipulation. *JAMA* 170:522–524, 1959.
22. Miller RG, Burton R: Stroke following chiropractic manipulation of the spine. *JAMA*

229:189–190, 1974.

23. Mueller S, Sahs AL: Brain stem dysfunction related to cervical manipulation. *Neurology* (*Minneap*) 26:547–550, 1976.

24. Pratt-Thomas HR, Berger KE: Cerebellar and spinal injuries after chiropractic manipulation. *JAMA* 133:600–603, 1947.

25. Schwartz GA: Posterior inferior cerebellar artery syndrome of Wallenberg after chiropractic manipulation. *Arch Intern Med* 97:352–354, 1956.

26. Smith RA, Estridge MN: Neurologic complications of head and neck manipulations. *JAMA* 182:528–531, 1962.

27. Braun IF, Pinto RS, DeFilipp GJ, Lieberman A, Pasternack P, Zimmerman RD: Brain stem infarction due to chiropractic manipulation of the cervical spine. *South Med J* 76:1507–1510, 1983.

28. Horn SW: The locked-in syndrome following chiropractic manipulation of the cervical spine. *Ann Emerg Med* 12:648–650, 1983.

29. Hope EE, Bodensteiner JB, Barnes P: Cerebral infarction related to neck position in an adolescent. *Pediatrics* 72:335–337, 1983.

30. Okawara S, Nibbelink D: Vertebral artery occlusion following hyperextension and rotation of the head. *Stroke* 5:640–642, 1974.

31. Jaskoviak PA: Complications arising from manipulation of the cervical spine. *J Manip Physiolog Ther* 3:213–220, 1980.

32. Kleynhans AM: Complications of and contraindications to spinal manipulative therapy. In Haldeman S (ed): *Modern Developments in the Principles and Practice of Chiropractic.* New York, Appleton-Century-Crofts, 1980, pp 359–384.

33. Kleynhans AM: Vascular changes occurring in the cervical musculocutaneous system. *J Can Chiropractic Assoc* 15:19–21, 1970.

34. Palmateer DC: Greater occipital-trigeminal syndrome. *J Clin Chiropractic* (arch ed), 46–48, Winter 1972.

35. Zeoli NJ: Anatomical and pathological considerations of the circle of Willis. *Dig Chiropractic Econ* 13:44–45, 1971.

36. Giles LGF: Vertebral-basilar artery insufficiency. *J Can Chiropractic Assoc* 22:112–117, 1977.

37. Dintenfass J: *Chiropractic—A Modern Way To Health.* New York, Pyramid Books, 1970.

38. Heistad DD, Marcus ML, Gross PM: Effects of sympathetic nerves on cerebral vessels in dog, cat and monkey. *Am J Physiol* 235:544–552, 1978.

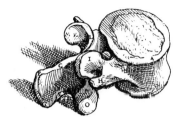

Chapter 10

Axoplasmic Aberration Hypothesis

*C*hiropractic researchers at the University of Colorado have made great strides in documenting and quantifying the effects of trauma on the neural mechanism of axoplasmic transport (AXT) (1–4). One of the few studies by chiropractic researchers other than those at the University of Colorado was conducted by Fernandez (5). The scientific community has given considerable emphasis to mechanisms of AXT (6–17). Researchers have shown that there are fast and slow or "bulk" AXT mechanisms and that AXT occurs in opposite directions along the nerve fiber (7–11, 16–23). In addition to proteins, glycoproteins, and neurotransmitters, constituents that are required for proper nerve growth and maintenance have been shown to be mobilized by AXT (9, 18–23).

Triano and Luttges (1) and other researchers at the University of Colorado have made discoveries that indicate that even moderate compression or intermittent irritation can significantly block or alter AXT in spinal nerves (2–4). Sjostrand et al. (24) have been able to demonstrate vagal sensitivity to AXT block. The *axoplasmic aberration* hypothesis, i.e., that AXT may be altered in certain cases in which the spinal nerve roots or spinal nerves are compressed or irritated by intervertebral subluxation, is discussed in light of these and similar studies.

A Unifying Transport Mechanism

The transport of axoplasmic components has been the focus of numerous investigations during the past decade. Weiss and Hiscoe (6) were the first to note that nerve growth might be influenced

121

by constituents of axoplasm. Studies have since confirmed their observations and shown that there is rapid or *fast axoplasmic transport* (FAXT) as well as "bulk flow" or slow AXT mechanisms that simultaneously carry a variety of constituents through nerves in probably all mammalian species (7, 8). Because the transport of these elements in neurons is not limited to the axon, Samson (7) has suggested that a more proper term would be neuroplasmic transport. In addition to FAXT and slow AXT, there is transport of constituents in both directions inside nerve fibers. Hence, *anterograde* or forward-moving products include those deemed important for nerve growth (9). Conversely, *retrograde* or backward-moving materials are transported from the nerve terminals to the cell bodies (9). Various researchers (12–15) have demonstrated chemicals that block AXT in an endeavor to determine a unifying concept that would explain the basis of its mechanism.

The intracellular movement in neurons appears to follow the same general principles that it follows in all eukaryotic cells (7). Basically, three primary areas have been explored with use of the electron microscope, AXT-blocking chemicals, and radioactive tracer (e.g., pulse-chase experiments). The three areas of the neuron that might provide mechanisms for transport of neuroplasmic constituents include the plasma membrane, tubular organelles (endoplasmic reticulum and microtubular channels), and fibrillar elements (actomyosin, microfilaments, neurofilaments, and microtubules) (7).

One of the proposed mechanisms for AXT takes into account the fact that actomyosin is found universally in eukaryotic cells (8). It has been shown that in these cells the actomyosin complex is responsible for nearly all of the intracellular and cellular movements. Because these units, known especially for their role in muscle fiber contraction, are also found in neurons, Allen (8) has suggested that they may perform a functional role in AXT. This is considered a unifying concept because it would explain that the movement seen in AXT is found throughout the animal kingdom. It is probable that at least the intracellular movements involving bulk cytoplasmic transport (slow AXT) are motivated by actomyosin (7).

A similar proposal has been based on the extensive studies of Ochs (10, 11, 16). It was found that injection of ^{3}H-leucine or ^{3}H-lysine into L7 dorsal nerve root ganglion or into the motoneuron region of the spinal cord resulted in a characteristic crest that was followed by a plateau of transported labeled axoplasmic constituents (10). The rate for FAXT was determined to be constant at 410 ± 50 mm/day regardless of nerve fiber size, diameter, and presence or absence of myelination. A wide variety of constituents, independent of their molecular weight, were found to move in this manner. Ochs (10, 11, 16), therefore, proposed a *sliding filament* hypothesis in which constituents bind to a *transport filament* which, in turn, is transported by connecting cross bridges (similar to actin/myosin) along the microtubules (MTs) and/or neurofilaments of the nerve fiber. It was explained that slow AXT actually involves materials exported into the nerve fibers later from some storage space or compartment within the cell body at a rate of 1 to 3 mm/day. Hence, it has been said tht slow AXT occurs because these constituents are released from the compartment over a period of time, which thus accounts for the plateau seen in these studies (10, 11, 16).

Samson (17) has agreed with the microtubule hypothesis, although his idea is that they bind directly to constituents with actomyosin cross bridges. He has stated that it is a unifying type of mechanism because MTs are found universally in the motile processes of flagella, sperm tails, and elsewhere in the cell. According to Samson, their location within the cell shows that they at least act as "guides" for AXT. Evidence shows that drugs that disrupt or have an affinity for MT protein subunits are also found to stop AXT, and this is further proof of their involvement (17).

Other mechanisms for AXT have been proposed, but it is beyond the scope of our discussion to review them all. The aforementioned mechanisms should suffice to give us an idea of the complexity and specificity that researchers have found in AXT (7-11, 16, 17). One concept presented early in the investigation of AXT was that both retrograde transport and anterograde transport occur. A brief discussion of this aspect of AXT is necessary in order to determine the implications of nerve compression.

Anterograde and Retrograde AXT

As previously mentioned, AXT has been demonstrated to occur both anterogradely and retrogradely. Anterograde movement has been shown to involve greater numbers of constituents and to be faster than retrograde AXT (anterograde FAXT occurs at a rate of 410 ± 50 mm/day, while retrograde FAXT occurs at a rate of 110 to 220 mm/day) (10, 11).

Anterograde movement of axoplasmic constituents has been shown to involve the transport of products important for nerve growth mechanisms (9). These constituents apparently are synthesized in the nerve cell bodies and moved by AXT to the neuron terminals proximodistally (9). There is now little question that embryonic sensory neurons depend on nerve growth factor (NGF) not only for growth but also for survival, at least *in vitro* (18). In addition, anterograde AXT is essential for transport of proteins and glycoproteins that maintain synaptic membranes and of other constituents of functional significance to the nerve endings (19). This role of AXT in supplying the *trophic* needs of tissue, even if only neural tissue, cannot be overemphasized. Bjoerklund et al. (20) have shown that transplants preincubated in a medium containing NGF are more densely and more rapidly innervated by adrenergic fibers. Moreover, preincubation of these transplants in media containing antibodies to NGF markedly impair the reinnervation of the transplant with adrenergic nerve fibers (20). Similarly, the substance P (a neurotransmitter) content of dorsal horns was shown to be affected by section of the peripheral processes of rat sciatic nerve (21). This was said to be the effect of neural degeneration and subsequent arrest of AXT (anterograde) (21). There is evidence that substance P is a transmitter for primary afferent fibers and specifically for nociceptive afferents in the substantia gelatinosa of the spinal cord (25, 26). These studies verify that anterograde AXT is an important, if not an essential, factor in the maintenance of the neuromuscular system.

Retrograde AXT involves materials that are transported from nerve terminals to the cell bodies. It has been shown that, in addition to other constituents, NGF is transported retrogradely (22, 23). NGF is taken up selectively into sympathetic neurons and is transported to the cell body where it apparently regulates the production of enzymes involved in transmitter synthesis; it has been demonstrated that nerve activity does not affect the AXT of NGF (27). NGF acts only on the neurons that transport it, and there is no evidence that NGF is released to act on extracellular sites (28). Treatment of newborn animals with antibodies to NGF has been shown to cause widespread sympathetic nervous system destruction (23). The retrograde transport of NGF is probably necessary for the development and maintenance of innervating adrenergic neurons (23). It can be seen that retrograde AXT—as well as anterograde AXT—is considered to play an important role in neuromuscular development as well as in maintenance.

Nerve Compression as a Factor in AXT

Studies have demonstrated that nerve compression may play a significant role in aberrant AXT. Although Ochs (29) has shown that compressive forces of 300 mm Hg block FAXT in sciatic nerve, it is known that lesser pressures can produce that result. Utilizing the ^{3}H-leucine isotope, Sjostrand et al. (24) was able to demonstrate that in sensory vagus nerve, ony 50 mm Hg pressure maintained for 2 hours caused FAXT block (30). This, of course, demonstrates the extreme susceptibility of AXT to compression trauma. This block was reversed within 1 day, whereas with greater pressures, longer recovery times were required (24, 30). In contrast to the susceptibility of nerve to AXT block by compression, studies have shown that much greater pressures are required in order to block nerve conduction (31–33). Apparently, among the most probable explanations for the mechanism of FAXT block by nerve compression is the possibility that local ischemia or changes in the ionic environment dramatically alter the normal AXT mechanism (29). This latter hypothesis is consistent with research that has demonstrated that alteration of the ionic balance within neurons can block FAXT (10, 11, 29).

Modern studies at the University of Colorado under the direction of Suh (1–4, 34–36) have thoroughly documented the protein composition of peripheral nerves in health and disease. Using modern electrophoretic and electrophysiologic techniques, Luttges et al. (2) have been able to more specifically analyze degenerative and regenerative events within the neuron. Their approach centered around the use of sodium dodecyl sulfate-polyacrylamide gel electrophoresis (SDS-PAGE) with subcellular fractionations. These researchers have identified more than 40 major protein bands by use of this system (2, 3) (Figure 10.1). These proteins were analyzed during nerve degeneration following various types of experimentally induced traumata including nerve crush, ligation, and section. In comparison with those in

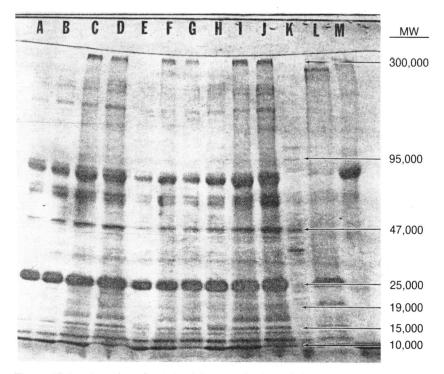

Figure 10.1.   Samples of proximal (*A* and *B*), distal (*C*), and control (*D*) sciatic nerve proteins following midthigh sciatic nerve ligation. Estimates of molecular weight (*MW*) are based on T_3 bacteriophage proteins (*K*) and autoradiographic techniques. Other samples relate to variations in extraction and centrifugation procedures, as well as to variations in the amount of protein being analyzed. Utilizing an SDS-PAGE system, Luttges and co-workers (2–4) were able to identify more than 40 major protein bands in mouse sciatic nerve (see text). (From Suh CH: Researching the fundamentals of chiropractic. In Suh CH (ed): *Proceedings of the 5th Annual Biomechanics Conference on the Spine.* Boulder, CO, University of Colorado, 1974, pp 1–52 (34).)

control nerves, some proteins exhibited increased composition and others exhibited decreased composition. The findings in one early study indicated that nerve conduction capacity varied in proportion to the apparent deterioration of nerve proteins (2). Another finding was that cut and ligation-type injuries produced more severe damage than did crush injuries.

In order to determine more precisely the damage involved with crush injuries, Luttges and Groswold (4) used fine forceps to crush a 2-mm area of mouse sciatic nerve. Electrophoretic and histologic examinations revealed only minimal discoloration and swelling in the sciatic nerve proximal to the zone of injury after 10 days. Distal to the injury, however, large decreases of some proteins (myelin glycoprotein and slow- and fast-migrating basic proteins (BP_{S1}, BP_{S2}, BP_{F1}, and BP_{F2}); S1 and F1 indicate slow and fast AXT, respectively) were noted along with obvious swelling and discoloration (Table 10.1). One interesting point was that for every 4 glycoprotein molecules, there were 2 BP_F and 1 BP_S that

Table 10.1. Characteristics of mouse protein following crush injury to sciatic nerve[a]

Degenerative characteristics	Regenerative characteristics
Proximal to midthigh crush	*Proximal and distal to midthigh crush*
By the tenth day, slight discoloration and slight edema; slight decrements of myelin glycoprotein and certain fast-migrating basic proteins	A. Decreased levels of certain slow-migrating basic proteins
Proximal and distal to midthigh crush	B. At 21 days, increments in some basic proteins distal to nerve crush and decrements in some proteins proximal to crush; myelin increases and concentrations of nuclear histones are evident at 35 days
A. By the 10 days, nuclear histones are discernible	C. Between 40 and 50 days, protein characteristics return to normal
B. By the thirtieth day, migration of certain fast-migrating basic proteins and histones	*Distal to midthigh crush*
C. Histones increase, then decrease in quantity	A. By 21 days, increased slow- and fast-migrating proteins and myelin glycoprotein
D. Increases of certain proteins during degeneration	B. At 21 days, protein of high molecular weight increases in quantity; other proteins show increments at this point also
Distal to midthigh crush	
By the tenth day, discoloration and edema; decrements of myelin glycoprotein and slow- and fast-migrating basic proteins	

[a] From Luttges MW, Groswald DE: Degenerative and regenerative characterizations in the proteins of mouse sciatic nerves. In Suh CH (ed): *Proceedings of the 7th Annual Biomechanics Conference on the Spine.* Boulder, CO, University of Colorado, 1976, pp 71–81 (4).

appeared to migrate as a unit. Luttges and his colleagues believed that this might be some type of axoplasmic functional unit. From a neurophysiologic viewpoint, these scientists appear to be well on the way to characterizing degenerative and regenerative events.

Discussion

As seen previously in Chapter 6, intervertebral subluxations may result in foraminal encroachment in all areas of the human spine. As was also seen, the likelihood of subsequent neural involvement is greatest in the cervical and lumbar regions where the diameter of spinal nerve in comparison with the intervertebral foramen is largest. Neurophysiologists have determined that nerve roots are highly susceptible to compression block but that spinal nerves are very resistant to block (31–33). This chapter has shown, however, that one highly important aspect of neuronal function is the delivery of constituents to various locations in the nerve cell by AXT. It has been demonstrated that vagus nerve is susceptible to AXT block when even minimal pressures are applied (50 mm Hg for 2 hours) (24, 30).

Another aspect of nerve injury, which has not been presented in this chapter, is the possibility of damaging the blood-nerve barrier (37). Scientists have shown, however, that even when pressures of 600 mm Hg are applied for 4 hours, they do not affect the blood-nerve barrier; consequently, this aspect of neuronal function has not been given attention (38).

Several important points should be kept in mind with regard to the effect of compression on neuronal function. Nerve conduction, axonal transport, and blood-nerve barrier are all affected by trauma. They differ, however, in susceptibility and reversibility and may be differentially affected (39). Although some researchers have found a correlation between regeneration and AXT, others have not (2, 4, 10, 40, 41). Hence, Cuenod (41) reported that AXT can recover in the absence of nerve regeneration and that block of AXT by colchicine does not cause nerve degeneration even after 6 weeks.

In their classical study of the role of mild, intermittent irritation of sciatic nerves of mice (by a Silastic implant) on conduction velocity as well as on chemical composition (via electrophoretic analysis), Triano and Luttges (1) found altered vascular composition of albumin and red blood cells. It may be assumed that these changes were due to alterations in AXT. The clinical implications of this finding include the possibility that many of the varied and diffuse descriptions of sciatic distributed pain, numbness, etc. may be the result of altered AXT and subsequent toxic levels of proteins in various portions of the nerve. Hence, the patient proudly proclaiming that, "Doctor, you must be helping; that pain is moving on down my leg," may be describing the process of reversal of AXT block. Obviously, it is too soon to make accurate predictions, but the evidence clearly demonstrates the relative susceptibility of nerve to AXT block or irritation, and this may indeed be one chemical basis for pain in many neuromuscular pain syndromes treated by the chiropractor.

These studies indicate that AXT is a specific and important mechanism for the maintenance, repair, and growth of the nervous system. They suggest that the clinical evaluation of damage to this mechanism may be impossible in light of our present understanding, since damage to AXT may occur with or without damage to nerve conduction and blood-nerve barrier. These studies would appear to confirm the axoplasmic aberration hypothesis, in that in those cases in which intervertebral subluxations do affect the spinal nerves or roots, AXT may certainly be altered with significant consequences.

Summary

Axoplasmic transport (AXT) mechanisms have been studied in some detail, and it is known that microtubules, actomyosin, and some transport filament may be involved (6–17). AXT is an important mechanism for the transfer of specific proteins, glycoproteins, other constituents, and NGF in the neuron (10, 11, 19–22). Although nerve conduction, AXT, and blood-nerve barrier respond differently to various insults, it is known that AXT is more susceptible to compression trauma (24, 29). It is concluded that the axoplasmic aberration hypothesis is valid in that when spinal nerves or roots are compressed or irritated by intervertebral subluxation, AXT may certainly be altered with significant consequences.

References

1. Triano JJ, Luttges MW: Nerve irritation: a possible model of sciatic neuritis. *Spine* 7:129–136, 1982.
2. Luttges MW, Kelly PT, Gerren RA; Degenerative changes in mouse sciatic nerves. electrophoretic and electrophysiologic characterization. *Exp Neurol* 50:706–733, 1976.
3. Kelly PT, Luttges MW: Electrophoretic separation of nervous system proteins on exponential gradient polyacrylamide gels. *J Neurochem* 24:1077–1079, 1975.
4. Luttges MW, Groswald DE: Degenerative and regenerative characterizations in the proteins of mouse sciatic nerves. In Suh CH (ed): *Proceedings of the 7th Annual Biomechanics Conference on the Spine.* Boulder, CO, University of Colorado, 1976, pp 71–81.
5. Fernandez JL: The transport of protein in nerves. *ACA J Chiropractic* 10:17–24, 1972.
6. Weiss P, Hiscoe HB: Experiments on the mechanism of nerve growth. *J Exp Zool* 107:315–395, 1948.
7. Samson F: Axonal transport: the mechanisms and their susceptibility to derangement; anterograde transport. In Korr IM (ed): *The Neurobiologic Mechanisms in Manipulative Therapy.* New York, Plenum, 1978, pp 291–309.
8. Allen RD: Some new insights concerning cytoplasmic transport. *Symp Soc Exp Biol* 8:15–26, 1974.
9. Warwick R, Williams P (eds): *Gray's Anatomy*, ed 35. Philadelphia, Saunders, 1973, p 773.
10. Ochs S: A brief review of material transport in nerve fibers. In Goldstein M (ed): *The Research Status of Spinal Manipulative Therapy.* Washington, DC, Government Printing Office, 1975, pp 189–196.
11. Ochs S, Chan SY, Worth R: Calcium and the mechanism of axoplasmic transport. In Korr IM (ed): *The Neurobiologic Mechanisms in Manipulative Therapy.* New York, Plenum, 1978, pp 359–367.
12. Bunt AH, Lund RD: Vinblastine induced blockage of orthograde and retrograde axonal transport of protein in retinal ganglion cells. *Exp Neurol* 45:288–297, 1974.
13. Shelanski ML, Taylor EW: Isolation of a protein subunit from microtubules. *J Cell Biol* 34:549–554, 1967.
14. Wilson L, Bamburg JR, Mizel SB, Grisham LM, Creswell KM: Interaction of drugs with microtubular proteins. *Fed Proc* 33:158–166, 1974.
15. Zweig MH, Chignell CF: Interaction of some colchicine analogs, vinblastine and podophyllotoxin with rat brain microtubular protein. *J Biochem Pharmacol* 22:2141–2150, 1973.
16. Ochs S: Characteristics and a model for fast axoplasmic transport in nerve. *J Neurobiol* 2:331–345, 1971.
17. Samson FE: Mechanism of axoplasmic transport. *J Neurobiol* 2:347–360, 1971.
18. Stach RW, Stach BM, West NR: Nerve fiber outgrowth from dorsal root ganglia: ion dependency of nerve growth factor action. *J Neurochem* 33:845–855, 1979.
19. Goodrum JF: Axonal transport and metabolism of ^{3}H fucose- and ^{35}S sulfate-labeled macromolecules in the rat visual system. *Brain Res* 176:255–272, 1979.
20. Bjoerklund A, Bjerre B, Steneri U: Has nerve growth factor a role in the regeneration of central and peripheral catecholamine neurons? In Fuxe K, Olson L, Zotterman Y (eds): *Dynamics of Regeneration and Growth in Neurons.* New York, Pergamon, 1974, pp 389–409.
21. Jessell T, Tsunoo A, Kanazawa I, Otsuka M: Substance P: depletion in the dorsal horn of rat spinal cord after section of the peripheral processes of primary sensory neurons. *Brain Res* 168:247–259, 1979.
22. Johnson EM, Blumberg HM, Costrini NV, Bradshaw RA: Reduction by reserpine of the

accumulation of retrogradely transported 125 nerve growth factor in sympathetic neurons. *Brain Res* 178:389–401, 1979.

23. Stoeckel K, Paravicini U, Thoenen H: Specificity of the retrograde axonal transport of nerve growth factor. *Brain Res* 76:413–421, 1974.

24. Sjostrand J, Rydevik B, Lundborg G, McLean WG: Impairment of intraneural microcirculation, blood nerve barrier and axonal transport in experimental nerve ischemia and compression. In Korr IM (ed): *The Neurobiologic Mechanisms in Manipulative Therapy.* New York, Plenum, 1978, pp 337–355.

25. Nakata Y, Kusaka Y, Segawa T: Supersensitivity to substance P after dorsal root section. *Life Sci* 24:1651–1654, 1979.

26. Piercey MF, Dobry PJK, Schroeder LA, Einspahr FJ: Behavioral evidence that substance P may be a spinal cord sensory neurotransmitter. *Brain Res* 210:407–412, 1981.

27. Lees G, Chubb I, Freeman C, Geffen L, Rush R: Effect of nerve activity on transport of nerve growth factor and dopamine β-hydroxylase antibodies in sympathetic neurones. *Brain Res* 214:186–189, 1981.

28. Hendry IA, Bonyhady R: Retrogradely transported nerve growth factor increases ornithine decarboxylase activity in rat superior cervical ganglia. *Brain Res* 200:39–45, 1980.

29. Ochs S: Energy metabolism and supply of P to the fast axoplasmic transport mechanism in nerve. *Fed Proc* 33:1049–1058, 1974.

30. Rydevik B, McLean WG, Sjostrand J, Lundborg G: Blockage of axonal transport induced by acute, graded compression of the rabbit vagus nerve. *J Neur Neurosurg Psychiatr* 43:690–698, 1980.

31. Aguayo A, Nair CPV, Midgley R: Experimental progressive compression neuropathy in the rabbit. *Arch Neurol* 24:358–364, 1971.

32. Rainer GW, Mayer J, Sadler TR, Dirks D: Effect of graded compression on nerve conduction velocity. *Arch Surg* 107:719–721, 1973.

33. Sharpless SK: Susceptibility of spinal roots to compression block. In Goldstein M (ed): *The Research Status of Spinal Manipulative Therapy.* Washington, DC, Government Printing Office, 1975, pp 155–161.

34. Suh CH: Researching the fundamentals of chiropractic. In Suh CH (ed): *Proceedings of the 5th Annual Biomechanics Conference on the Spine.* Boulder, CO, University of Colorado, 1974, pp 1–52.

35. MacGregor RJ: A model for reticular-like networks: ladder nets, recruitment fuses, and sustained responses. *Brain Res* 41:345–363, 1972.

36. MacGregor RJ, Oliver RM: A general-purpose electronic model for arbitrary configurations of neurons. *J Theor Biol* 38:527–538, 1973.

37. Kolber AR, Bagnell CR, Krigman MR, Hayward J, Morell P: Transport of sugars into microvessels isolated from rat brain: a model for the blood-brain barrier. *J Neurochem* 33:419–432, 1979.

38. Sjostrand J: Discussion. In Korr IM (ed): *The Neurobiologic Mechanisms in Manipulative Therapy.* New York, Plenum, 1978, pp 369–373.

39. Sjostrand J: Discussion. In Korr IM (ed): *The Neurobiologic Mechanisms in Manipulative Therapy.* New York, Plenum, 1978, pp 357–358.

40. Spencer PS: Reappraisal of the model for 'bulk axoplasmic flow'. *Nature New Biol* 240:283–285, 1972.

41. Cuenod M: Contributions of axoplasmic transport to synaptic structures and functions. *Int J Neurosci* 4:77–87, 1972.

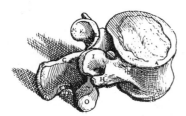

Chapter 11

Somatoautonomic Reflex Hypothesis

The most comprehensive review of the effects of aberrant so-matoautonomic reflexes in humans was perhaps that reported recently by various scientists attending a workshop on "Neuro-biologic Mechanisms in Manipulative Therapy" at Michigan State University (1). These scientists agreed that somatoautonomic reflexes affect a wide variety of functions in humans. *Somatoautonomic reflexes* may be defined as autonomic responses initiated by the transmission of signals from somatic afferent fibers located in the dermatomes. The principal focus of the workshop with regard to somatoautonomic reflexes was whether or not these reflexes are subject to derangement and what may be the clinical effects of such derangement.

It will be recalled from Chapter 8 that spinal fixation (SF) has been the subject of experimental investigation by scientists as well as by chiropractors and osteopaths. In Chapter 8, the fixation hypothesis is discussed in terms of lessened mobility within the vertebral motor unit, soft tissue involvement, aberrant neural reflexes including somatic afferent bombardment of dorsal horn cells, and resultant segmental facilitation. Clinical as well as experimental evidence of the SF is presented and discussed in light of what is known about those nervous system receptors and pathways in the spinal cord which may be involved. The conclusion reached is that the noxious or nociceptive (painful) impulses evoked from such a lesion predictably would have some influence on normal somatoautonomic pathways.

Chiropractic and osteopathic researchers have acknowledged for some time that spinal fixations can cause somatic afferent bombardment of dorsal horn cells that may alter normal autonomic reflexes or may evoke abnormal autonomic reflexes (2–9). This mechanism we will term the *somatoautonomic reflex* (SAR) hypothesis. A review of osteopathic experimental studies from 1914 to the present indicates that much has been shown about somatoautonomic reflexes and about the effects of SAR aberration (10–29). Further evidence regarding the SAR hypothesis is gained by a review of clinical studies conducted by medical doctors and doctors of osteopathy. The neural pathways involved in mediating the SF-SAR response are described in Chapter 8. The validity of the SAR hypothesis is discussed in light of the clinical and experimental evidence cited in the present chapter.

Osteopathic Experimental Studies

From 1914 until 1936, the A. T. Still Research Institute in Chicago performed investigations of vertebral lesions and their effects on the spines of cats, dogs, rats, rabbits, and guinea pigs. The effects of spinal lesions on blood chemistry, urine, gastric secretions, glandular tissues, vascular reflexes, tissue fluids, the progeny of lesioned animals, motility of the gastrointestinal tract, and many other body functions were measured cytologically, histologically, and morphologically, and the results in these lesioned animals were subsequently compared with those in matched unlesioned control animals. The data were massive and comprised the first scientific evidence that somatic dysfunction (i.e., spinal fixation, intervertebral subluxation) can result in pathophysiological changes in various body systems (10–29).

Before a review of osteopathic experimental research is begun, it is necessary to define what osteopaths then called the "osteopathic lesion" and what they now refer to as an area of "somatic dysfunction" (see Chapter 3). These terms denote a spinal lesion that is identifiable by x-ray, palpation, and corresponding visceral disturbances recognized in experimental animals on autopsy and in humans by laboratory diagnostic procedures (10). Identification of the osteopathic lesion by x-ray required either positive findings of edema or fibrosis or findings of an actual bony maladjustment (most analogous to an intervertebral subluxation). Palpation in these experiments was performed by more than one investigator acting independently. For determination of the positive finding of an osteopathic lesion, more than one investigator was required to identify the same area of bony maladjustment and/or localized tension due to fibrosis, edema, and muscular splinting and contraction. "Muscular contraction" was recognized by increased tonus of spinal muscles or by localized "knots" or "strings" in irregularly contracted muscles of the deeper spinal layers (see definition of muscle spasm in Chapter 8). Palpation often revealed hypersensitivity and rigidity which provided further corroboration of a lesion when identified. An animal was labeled as "lesioned" only when independent investigators identified the same lesion at the same vertebral level.

Among some of the earlier studies performed by osteopaths were projects designed to determine the effects of lower cervical and upper dorsal lesions on blood pressure and amplitude of heart beat. In one such study, Deason and Doron (11) induced lesions in this area of the spine by rotation and traction of the cephalic end of 9 dogs and 2 cats while the lower cervical and upper dorsal spines were fixed. Consequently, most lesions appeared in the lower cervical spine. All animals were previously anesthetized with ether by deep and constant tracheal cannula (viz., a tube inserted deep into the trachea). Respiration was monitored, the sciatic nerve was sectioned and stimulated by medium faradic current, and blood pressure was taken from the carotid or the femoral artery with a manometer. As had been established in previous experiments, stimulation applied to the central end of the sciatic nerve caused an increase in heart rate, respiration, and blood pressure. The average rate of increase in blood pressure was 6.6 mm above normal. After the animals were lesioned, however, the same stimulation resulted not in an increase but in a decrease in blood pressure below the normal rate in 9 of 11 animals. The average decline was 5.3 mm below normal. The heart rate did not significantly decline. The authors concluded that an acute lesion will affect the normal spinal sympathetic reflexes. This study was among the first to document the effects of spinal lesions on somatosympathetic neural pathways.

In another early study, Pengra and Alexander (12) determined the effects of spondylotherapy and osteopathic stimulation on the secretion of urine in 11 dogs. The animals were operated on after anesthesia with ether (by tracheal cannula), and both ureters were cannulated (the urine was collected in graduated test tubes).

Respiration, blood pressure, and heart rate were monitored and allowed to become rhythmical following the operation and throughout the experiments. Several counts were taken between 10-minute intervals (to ascertain the exact rate of normal urine flow). At this point, some of the animals received spondylotherapy (concussion of the region of the spine innervating the kidneys, or the dorsal 12 and 13 vertebrae, with a light hammer and rubber cord as a percussion pad). This group acted as a control, to determine whether nonspecific stimulation could affect urine flow. In the experimental group, osteopathic manipulation was applied by lateral rotation and by making fixed points of the spinous processes of two adjacent vertebrae (in the area of the spine innervating the kidneys). In the control group, percussion alone was found to have no effect on urine flow in any animal. In the group receiving specific osteopathic stimulation, however, the rate of urine secretion increased dramatically, from a 20% to a more than 100% rise in some animals. Blood pressure and respiration did not change in these animals; so it was determined that the increased function of the kidneys in these animals was due to either specific vasomotor or secretory (trophic) nerve fibers (which were influenced without changing general systemic vasomotor activity). The animals were monitored for signs of infection; none occurred during the experiments (usually lasting several hours or longer). Perhaps most interesting is the finding that the spinal treatments were specific in effect, not significantly affecting other metabolic systems.

In those and other early osteopathic studies, exact measurement of osteopathic treatment must have varied from animal to animal. In fact, there has never been an accurate method in either osteopathy or chiropractic for delivering spinal thrusts of the same depth, speed, and direction, because until recently all such treatments or adjustments were performed by hand. This is an important variable to consider. Even if machines had been developed for use on animals and in the clinic, the biologic response of each individual is still a variable that must be considered. In all fairness to these researchers, however, it appears that they did their homework. In each study, numerous variables were monitored or controlled; unfortunately, it is beyond the scope of this text to detail all such considerations.

By 1917, Hoskins (13) had performed preliminary studies on

the effects of barium meal combined with other foods after various fluoroscopic examinations in dogs, cats, guinea pigs, rabbits, and white rats. It was found that cats enjoyed a salmon-barium meal and fluoroscopic examination with no observeable side effects. These animals actually purred during such examinations. By minimizing x-radiation and the amount of the meal, Hoskins was able to monitor motility of the gastrointestinal tract in both lesioned and control animals until the meal had completely left the colon. The average time for passage of the meal through all 27 healthy animals was 26 hours 46.2 minutes. After establishment of a lesion in the dorsal-lumbar spine (and monitoring of the lesion for 10 to 14 days), however, the average time for passage of the same meal in the same animals was 30 hours 17.1 minutes. Some of the animals were utilized as controls and remained nonlesioned but were reexamined 10 to 14 days later along with the lesioned animals. The lesions were monitored by x-ray, and the conclusion was reached that a dorsal-lumbar lesion had a definite effect of retarding gastrointestinal tract motility. Additionally, the author noted that many animals in the series had to be rejected after contracting pneumonia; interestingly, the lesioned animals had a greater tendency to contract this disease, although no conclusions could be drawn due to the limited number of test animals.

By the 1930s, osteopathic research methods had become even more definitive, and under the guidance of its director L. Burns, the A. T. Still Research Institute published *Bulletin 7*, which contained several papers documenting reflex pathophysiology of the osteopathic lesion.

Two studies by Burns (14, 15) showed that lesions of the fifth thoracic and adjacent vertebrae tended to result in increased acidity of the gastric juice and a tendency to gastric ulceration. Interestingly, lesions of the seventh thoracic vertebra resulted in decreased acidity of the gastric juice and atony of the gastric wall. Dozens of guinea pigs were utilized in these experiments which extended for months; in each case, control animals were utilized in addition to the experimental animals.

In yet another series on gastric acidity, osteopathic researchers noted that rapid vibratory movements of deep spinal muscles in male lesioned or nonlesioned cats will interfere markedly with normal gastric secretions (16). Physiologists have since documented that the nervous signals that cause gastric secretion originate in the dorsal motor nuclei of the vagi (in the medulla oblongata) (30). These signals affect the stomach by way of vagal nerves; this explains why one medical treatment for peptic ulcer is vagotomy. Peptic ulcers generally disappear within 1 week of the operation; unfortunately, for many patients the ulcer returns and gastric atony develops immediately following such surgery (30, 31). These findings would tend to support the osteopathic data, since somatosympathetic pathways, once excited, could inhibit the action of the parasympathetic nervous system (and hence the vagus nerve).

In another series of remarkable experiments, osteopathic researchers examined the gastric juice in 40 young rabbits that had one lesioned parent (17). From 2 to 4 months following birth, these animals were sacrificed by a single sharp blow to the back of the head. Immediately, the stomachs were removed and the titrated contents were compared with the contents from 20 normal young rabbits with normal parents. The average gastric acidity in the group with one lesioned parent was 8% free hydrochloric acid (HCl), with a range of 0% to 13%. The average gastric acidity in the control rabbits with normal parents was 36% free HCl, with a range of 33% to 38%. This statistically significant difference appears to suggest that the effects of an intervertebral lesion on gastric acidity in progeny is very marked.

Equally fantastic results were found in one renal study in which 17 Peruvian long-haired guinea pigs from normal stock were individually examined for lesions by independently acting investigators (18). No lesions were found in any of these animals. Subsequently, 12 of the guinea pigs were given lesions (spinous process right, right articular process caudad, and left transverse process cephalad) at the dorsal 12 and 13 vertebral levels. These researchers called this displacement a "subluxation." Five guinea pigs were utilized as nonlesioned controls. The guinea pigs were killed at various times following the onset of the lesion (from 1 hour to 1 year later).

Five of the lesioned pigs were matched at autopsy with the five controls who had not been lesioned (18). In every case, independent researchers correctly separated the lesioned from the nonlesioned animals at autopsy, although they had not been told which guinea pigs were experimental and which were controls. In 1 guinea pig sacrificed 1 hour following inducement of the lesion, there was an abnormal amount of erythrocytes crowding the blood vessels of the kidneys. In addition, the epithelium of the glomeruli showed a lack of differentiation. A control guinea pig also sacrificed at this time showed no such changes. In guinea pigs killed 24 and 48 hours following initiation of the lesion, diapedesis of both red and white blood cells was visible in various areas; there was also evidence of cloudy swelling in the glomerular epithelium and slight desquamation of the tubular epithelium. Pigs killed 4 and 7 days following the inducement of the lesion showed more pronounced cloudy swelling affecting the entire kidneys. The lymph in these animals contained occasional fatty globules, and some casts and many leukocytes were noted in the tubules. None of these changes were evident in the control guinea pig sacrificed during this period. Three other guinea pigs were sacrificed 1 month, 3 months, and 1 year, respectively, following onset of their lesions. Round cell infiltration was seen several months following the lesion. Blood vessels were crowded, and hemorrhages per diapedesis, cloudy swelling and fatty degeneration were found to about the same degree in these animals as were found in animals sacrificed earlier. Some hyaline and granular casts were noted. One year following initiation of the lesion, however, fatty degeneration was more pronounced. Cloudy swelling, hemorrhages per diapedesis, and connective tissue overgrowth indicated that pathology of a more serious nature had occurred. Apparently, scar-like areas of connective tissue marked the sites of earlier minute hemorrhages. These casts were less abundant than those seen earlier. These findings were compared with data taken from studies on white rats, rabbits, cats, and dogs. The authors concluded that intervertebral lesions at the dorsal 12 and 13 vertebral levels affected the metabolism of the renal epithelium and the circulation through the kidneys. It is noteworthy that these animals appeared to function normally from the moment that they were lesioned to the time of their death. All pathophysiology in these animals was of a renal microscopic nature.

Studies at the A. T. Still Research Institute also linked lesions to changes in blood constituents, urine, and tissue fluids by use of similar methods (19–21). These researchers noted that urine and tissue fluid abnormalities occurred in relation to the amount of pathologic activity in the various organs of these lesioned

animals. Hence, lesions of the occiput, atlas, and axis were associated with circulation through the pituitary. The urine abnormalities that then developed as a result of the moderate increase in
pleural, pericardial, peritoneal, and scrotal fluids were seen as
subnormal excretion of water and as excretion of urine with a
high specific gravity (19). These animals showed weight increases
beyond normal and control limits, due to increased extracellular
fluid levels. Although the kidneys showed no signs of pathology
on a macroscopic or microscopic level, the hearts of these animals
showed signs of muscular weakness, and low arterial blood pressure was associated with an increase in extracellular fluids that
had caused slight cardiac dilation. At the time of these studies,
the researchers apparently had no idea of the pathogenesis of
these phenomena (other than that vertebral lesions had been a
factor in the etiology). Today, we can note a striking similarity
between the pathogenesis of this condition and the pathophysiology of increased antidiuretic hormone secretion (by the neurohypophysis) (32).

Similarly, conditions of local acidosis were noted in cats, rabbits,
and guinea pigs in various tissues following initiation of a dorsal
10 vertebral lesion (20). Results of autopsy of these animals, when
matched with the results of autopsy of nonlesioned controls,
showed that vertebral lesions caused a marked decrease in alka-
linity in tissues of the small, deep spinal muscles in the area
around the affected vertebrae. Furthermore, viscera affected by
the segmental distribution of the sympathetic nerves involved
with the lesion showed a state of acidosis, moderate edema,
minute hemorrhages, and other evidences of circulatory disturbance. These findings corroborated earlier studies showing microscopic renal pathology as a result of renal circulatory disturbances,
as previously mentioned (18, 20).

Perhaps the most amazing and interesting of all osteopathic
studies lending validity to the SAR hypothesis was performed in
1931 by Cherrill et al. (21, 22). In a series of experiments on
animals, which were correlated with findings from human clinical
studies, these researchers reported on "costogenic anemia" and
other abnormal blood conditions in which lesions of either the
corresponding rib and/or the vertebra were involved. Lesions in
these animals were associated with poikilocytosis and anisocytosis
at equal levels, low hemoglobin counts (as much as 40% below

normal), and small red blood cells that were vacuolated and sometimes nucleated (21). Immature forms of blood cells were abundant, including plasma cells, mast cells, and basophilic and eosinophilic polymorphonuclear cells (all present in varying degrees of immaturity). A mechanism was hypothesized whereby the lesions affected the sympathetic tone of the vessels supplying the involved red bone marrow. This caused a decrease in circulation to the marrow and, hence, gave rise to "costogenic anemia." Secondary anemias were also demonstrated in test animals when vertebral lesions caused gastric ulcers, hyperchlorhydria, hypochlorhydria, gastric atony, and gastroptosis. These conditions impaired digestion and absorption and left these animals anemic and thin, as would be expected. When the blood conditions described previously were seen in test animals with corresponding vertebral and/or costal lesions and were not seen in control animals, it was suggested that the lesions had caused a decrease in circulation through the red bone marrow and that this was the mechanism whereby anemia had been produced (21).

Experimental and control rabbits matched for weight, age, nutrition, environment, and genetic background were sacrificed together by identical methods in one study, to determine the effects of lower cervical and upper thoracic lesions on leukocytes in nasal and pharyngeal membranes (21). Ten months after a second thoracic lesion was produced a rabbit designated as HT7 was sacrificed along with a control animal designated as HT9 (these animals happened to be twins). Following removal of the mandible, the throat could be easily viewed in these experiments; in HT7, the pharyngeal and nasal membranes were swollen and thickened. Pouch-like folds appeared to be small nasal polyps, which were especially abundant in the nasal membranes. The blood vessels were crowded with cells; the plasma layer was seemingly invisible. Goblet cells were ten times as abundant in this animal as in the normal control animal (HT9). Lymphoid elements were hypertrophied, and hyaline cells were twice as numerous in arterioles as in veins. What is significant is that in the control animal these changes were not evident. Subsequent tests with 5 cats (including 1 control) and 6 experimental guinea pigs verified these findings (21). Further blood cell examinations were completed in 5 lesioned and 5 control cats, rabbits, and guinea pigs (21). In each case, 1 control and 1 experimental animal were sacrificed together; these were matched for age, size, heredity, and sex as well as other factors. The lymphocyte counts (viz., lymphocytes per cubic millimeter of blood) in the lesioned animals were 16% to 22% above the normal counts in control animals. Upper thoracic lesions were involved in these cases. If the lesion was not produced by accident, the spinous process was diverted toward the left, and the transverse process was diverted cephalad in each of these experiments. These experiments, according to researchers (21), left no doubt that vertebral lesions could result in changes in blood constituents and in the lymphocyte count.

Studies by Tweed (23) apparently documented the effects of vertebral lesions at the twelfth thoracic level on the suprarenals and the adrenals; in addition, changes in the thyroid were seen with lesions of the seventh cervical through third thoracic levels, and changes in the pancreas (especially in the islets of Langerhans) were induced by lesions at the levels of dorsal 8 through 10. Dozens of guinea pigs and rabbits were fed high-, normal-, or low-carbohydrate diets. Some were subjected to various lesions, but many had lesions of unknown origin prior to the experiment (these lesions were, nevertheless, identified by x-ray and palpation). Others were utilized as controls. All animals were fasted for 1 day prior to being sacrificed. Following a sharp blow to the head, a syringe previously rinsed with potassium oxalate solution was thrust through the chest wall into the heart. Generally, 6 to 9 cc of blood were withdrawn and were placed in a bottle containing some potassium oxalate crystals. The stomach was also immediately removed for gastric analysis; tissues of the various organs (thyroid, suprarenals, pancreas, etc.) were prepared for slides. Tweed found that blood sugar in normal control high-carbohydrate-diet guinea pigs varied from 100 to 125 mg/100 cc of blood. Blood sugar in the lesioned high-carbohydrate-diet guinea pigs, however, varied greatly from 82 to 166 mg/100 cc of blood. In the progeny of the lesioned high-carbohydrate-diet guinea pigs, the blood sugar varied even more, from 20 to 200 mg/100 cc of blood. Similar findings in the low-carbohydrate-diet control and lesioned pigs and in the high-carbohydrate-diet control and lesioned rabbits appeared to verify that various vertebral lesions may exert a marked influence on blood sugar levels. These lesions were nearly all in the dorsal-lumbar spine; other lesions in the cervical-dorsal spine were associated with marked changes in thyroid anatomy (including hemorrhages and evidence of circulatory changes). In all cases, the lesioned animals were matched with controls on the same diet for age, heredity, and time and technique of death. Microscopic examination of the islets of Langerhans and other pancreatic tissues in animals with corresponding vertebral lesions showed signs of atrophy, connective tissue proliferation, granulator degeneration, and hemorrhagic areas, especially in the cells of external secretion. These signs of circulatory deficiency were found in varying degrees and only in animals with corresponding lesions. When the suprarenals were involved, severe hemorrhages could be obviously seen, especially in the medulla; congestion in the cells of secretion could also be noted. Another sign of suprarenal involvement was connective tissue proliferation, which was marked in some cases. These same tissues appeared to be normal or to vary only slightly in all control animals. Urinalysis verified traces and high amounts of sugar in animals whose blood had indicated the same. Tweed (23) suggested that the only probable explanation for these findings was that circulation to these glands was affected by vertebral lesions at the corresponding spinal levels. Once circulation became aberrant, the glands could no longer properly regulate blood sugar levels or function normally.

Conclusions

Osteopathic experimental studies have documented to a convincing degree that various vertebral lesions in animals can markedly affect the circulation in several important glands and organs and can cause associated microscopic pathologies and degenerative abnormalities (10–29). According to these researchers, the mechanism to explain these effects is that vertebral lesions affect the circulation of the various organs by way of the sympathetic nerves that control constriction (tone) of blood vessels, especially those of the viscera. These somatosympathetic pathways apparently become routes for aberrant neural transmission when they are affected adversely by spinal fixation (see Chapter 8).

Clinical Studies

Of course, the true test of any hypothesis gained by experimental research is the successful application of that hypothesis in clinical practice. For nearly a century, chiropractors and osteopaths have utilized the SAR hypothesis to explain their clinical results, which have been impressive enough to sustain both professions and to encourage their progress. Obviously, many of these practitioners did not know or even care to know the name of this hypothesis. Nevertheless, when a chiropractor spoke of "bones pinching nerves" and "causing dis-ease" he or she was referring in broad terms to this phenomenon and to the neurodystrophic hypothesis described in Chapter 12. Osteopaths and chiropractors, however, have not been the only practitioners to describe and apply this hypothesis in the clinic.

Medical doctors Ussher (33, 34) and Wills and Atsatt (35) performed initial investigations of the "viscerospinal syndrome" in the 1930s. They reported 400 instances of this syndrome in a time span of several years. These investigators ruled out visceral pathologies in certain patients who reported visceral symptomatology. In these patients, definite orthopedic and roentgenologic findings of scoliosis and short-leg phenomena were reported. Furthermore, orthopedic correction of the scolioses, kyphoses, and lordoses—by utilization of heel lifts, physiotherapy, and supports and muscle training—resulted in relief or cure of the symptomatology in every case. This led these investigators to the conclusion that pathologic changes in spinal structure cause physiologic disturbances in the area of involved neurologic distribution. These researchers did not perform the basic research necessary to elucidate the exact neuronal pathways. Ussher, however, did propose the following hypothesis (33):

> It may be that physiopathologic changes in these spinal structures actually produce an inhibition of sympathetic impulses. In turn this inhibition may allow parasympathetic tone to predominate, resulting in what appears to be an actual parasympathetic rather than sympathetic action on the viscera.

Ussher (33, 34) has implicated both spinal nerve irritation and proprioceptive insult at the spinal level as probable factors in the initiation of this aberrant somatosympathetic reflex. He also believed that noxious impulses from the skin and dorsal musculature in an area of postural distortion could cause this reflex. Subjective and clinical findings that Ussher (33, 34) as well as Wills and Atsatt (35) associated with this syndrome included severe pain in various viscera, severe asthmatic attacks, bronchial asthma, symptoms of angina, esophageal spasm (documented by barium fluoroscopic examination of the esophagus), pylorospasm and other gastrointestinal complaints, marked constipation, painful and frequent micturation, and a host of other conditions. A careful medical investigation of each patient's complaint was made. Blood and urinalysis tests, fluoroscopic examinations, and radiographic examinations were utilized following accepted medical procedures to establish a correct diagnosis. These investigators determined that in each case, the viscerospinal syndrome was involved and that some degree of relief of the complaints or complete cure was achieved by correction of the spinal abnormalities. What is significant is that these were highly respected and qualified medical researchers presenting these data in major medical journals (33–35).

Murphy and Wilson (36) performed a study on patients with asthmatic bronchitis in 1925 in an effort to establish the value of osteopathic manipulative therapy. The Massachusetts Medical Society sponsored the study as part of an investigation of osteopathy and chiropractic. All 20 patients who were chosen had suffered nearly continuous attacks of asthma. All had failed to respond to vaccine therapy and had responded minimally to adrenalin injections. Instead of determining whether each patient had an osteopathic lesion, the investigators assumed that one existed at the fourth and fifth dorsal level (the segments presumed to be responsible for sympathetic nerve supply to the bronchial tubes and, hence, circulation). These patients were treated with from 10 to 70 osteopathic manipulations. No control patients were utilized to assess the psychosomatic involvement. Fifteen of 20 patients experienced at least some degree of temporary relief and 5 reported no change. Six of the 15 who reported relief of symptoms were very much improved (90% to 100%) and another 4 reported noticeable improvement (50% to 75%). No conclusions were drawn by the authors, but it is noteworthy that even without locating the exact osteopathic lesion, these investigators were able to treat the area of the spine segmentally associated with the visceral disturbance and to achieve significant results in 75% of these patients on whom medical treatments had previously failed.

Pottenger (37) concurred with Ussher that while there are no sympathetic sensory nerves per se, there are afferent somatic nerves that course through the sympathetic system and originate in the posterior horn of the cord. Thus, he envisioned (35)

> . . . a continuous stream of impulses coming to the cord from the somatic structures, which express themselves reflexly both in other somatic structures and in visceral structures.

His own observations and studies indicated the presence of both somatovisceral and viscerosomatic reflexes (37–39). For example, he studied the reflex effects of tuberculosis in a number of patients and found it to cause various aberrant reflexes. These resulted in a variety of secondary conditions: atrophy of the facial muscles, mucous membrane of the nose, and pharynx (mediated through the vagus and hypoglossal cranial nerves), atrophy of the tongue (also mediated through the vagus and hypoglossal nerves), and atrophy of the larynx (mediated through the laryngeal nerves). He was able to demonstrate increased tension and degeneration of the tongue and facial muscles as a result of chronic inflammation of the lung. He found reflex relationships between the lung and other viscera mediated by the vagus nerve, and he recognized the segmental relationship of sympathetically mediated viscerosomatic and somatovisceral reflexes. In other studies, this recognized medical pathologist and author of *Symptoms of Visceral Disease* noted vagally mediated somatovisceral reflexes which resulted in asthma and bronchitis; he suggested the possibility of this reflex in pulmonary collapse (acute pulmonary atelectasis) (37–39).

Modern osteopathic studies have brought application of the SAR hypothesis up to the highest standards of clinical science. Rogers and Rogers (40) in 1976 showed that in ischemic heart disease with angina pectoris and transient spasm of the coronary arteries, manipulation is of value in correcting the function of the autonomic nervous system. This, in turn, influenced the cellular metabolism and vasomotor dynamics of the coronary arteries. The authors reviewed two of their cases in which osteopathic manipulative therapy was shown by angiography and electrocardiography to produce improvement. These authors challenged the idea that atherosclerotic phenomena are responsible for both angina pectoris and myocardial infarction. They produced positive results that suggest that autoregulatory control of coronary artery flow was of principal importance in meeting the increased metabolic needs of the myocardium.

In a study of patients with chronic obstructive pulmonary disease, Miller (41) has shown that osteopathic manipulative therapy may be of value in increasing various lung capacities. In addition to the usual battery of medical tests, these patients were measured for blood gas tension and pulmonary function including lung volume, diffusion, maximum voluntary ventilation, vital capacity, FEV_1, and FEV_2, and midexpiratory flow rate. Forty-four patients with chronic obstructive pulmonary disease were divided into two groups: a control group that received only standard medical therapy and an experimental group that received medical therapy and specific osteopathic manipulation. The pulmonary function studies after treatment revealed that blood gas tension in both groups remained unchanged. The mean vital capacity (nearly identical for both groups before the study), however, improved 0.5 liters in the manipulated group as opposed to a slight 0.1 liter improvement in the control group. This improvement was not considered statistically significant ($p > 0.05$) because of the small numbers of patients involved in the study. The vital capacity, residual volume, and forced expiratory volume increased in the control group at about the same ratio. Subjective improvement, however, was very dramatic. Ninety-two percent of the patients who received osteopathic manipulation reported definite subjective improvement in their physical work capacity. This indicated that somatosympathetic pathways were involved in pulmonary pathology or at least in increasing lung capacities once such pathology had become chronic. A review of modern chiropractic research supporting the SAR hypothesis may be found in Chapter 13 under the heading, "Chiropractic Treatment of Organic Disorders."

Discussion

From a review of osteopathic experimental studies performed in this century, it seems that these researchers were trying to conclude that vertebral lesions can cause practically any of a number of experimental pathologies of a functional nature. In fact, if indeed the results that these investigators achieved are accurate, it must be said that at the very least these "lesions" produced significant results.

Alterations in blood chemistry were associated with the effects of lesions on sympathetic tone to blood vessels that supply red bone marrow (21, 22). These effects included alteration of lymphocyte count as well as production of immature plasma cells by marrow. DePace and Webber (42) demonstrated that lumbar sympathetic stimulation results in stimulation of bone marrow to release reticulocytes and neutrophils. Others (43) have previously demonstrated that autonomic tone can have a neurovascular effect on bone marrow function.

Gastric acidity was the focus of several osteopathic studies (14–17). There is now ample evidence to suggest that somatoautonomic pathways (cutaneovisceral) may certainly affect gastrointestinal tract function (44–48). Likewise osteopathic evidence that lesions can affect certain parameters of heart function is substantiated by recent findings that somatoautonomic pathways (cutaneovisceral) may affect heart rate by altering vagal activity (11, 45–47, 49–51). In fact, current research has indicated that autonomic imbalance plays a strong role in the pathogenesis of spontaneous angina (excluding Prinzmetal's angina) (52). Matoba et al. (52) were able to demonstrate complete relief of chest pain in 13 of 13 patients with angina who had augmented levels of autonomic activity and positive stress testing, by giving calcium antagonists orally. This finding supports the work of Rogers and Rogers (40) in that it suggests an autonomic role for pathogenesis of angina. An animal model of sudden infant death syndrome (SIDS) showed that epileptogenic activity correlated with changes in cardiovascular function and autonomic cardiac neural discharge and that, before death, an imbalance was found between sympathetic and parasympathetic cardiac neural discharges (see also Chapter 7) (53). Investigators (54, 55) have shown too that sympathectomy and injuries to the peripheral and autonomic innervating nerves as well as neuroexcitation can enhance the development of arteriosclerosis.

Early investigations into the role of vertebral lesions and various pulmonary disorders have been similarly substantiated in part by modern research (33–39, 41, 45–47, 49, 50, 56). For example, current research on the mechanisms of allergic asthma and allergic rhinitis indicates a role for autonomic imbalance in the pathogenesis of the disease (57). Hence, researchers have found that there is a basic defect in patients with asthma and that this defect causes increased secretion of pulmonary mast cell mediators (e.g., histamine). This increased secretion, then, leads to an alteration in autonomic activity, in autonomic receptors, or in effector mechanisms. Kaliner et al. (30) were able to demonstrate autoantibodies to beta receptors in 24 patients with seasonal or perennial allergic rhinitis. These patients were found to have beta adrenergic hyporeactivity and cholinergic hypersensitivity. Since beta adrenergic agonists modulate the allergen-induced release of mast cell mediators that produce the inflammatory response, autoantibodies to these receptors would be expected to promote an allergic response. It is known that the autonomic activity is not the primary defect, since administration of beta blockers to normal subjects does not make them asthmatic (57). A role for stress and autonomic imbalance (including the role of spinal stress from a vertebral lesion), however, could be expected to enhance an allergic response (see Chapter 12). Either increased cholinergic or alpha adrenergic activity or decreased beta adrenergic activity in the smooth muscles of the bronchial airways would be expected to enhance an asthmatic episode (56). It is easy to see, therefore, that some combination of spinal stress with somatoautonomic aberrant reflexes and superimposed genetic predisposition to asthma may be responsible for especially marked episodes of the disease and may account for the mechanism whereby chiropractic manipulation may be of benefit in its treatment.

The role of somatic sensations causing alterations of autonomic function has been dramatically demonstrated by Ekman et al. (31). These investigators were able to demonstrate that autonomic activity distinguishes between positive and negative emotions and even distinguishes among different types of negative emotion. Such a powerful role for the autonomic nervous system had not previously been expected. In their study, it was found that constructing facial prototypes of emotion muscle by muscle resulted in a more powerful autonomic response than did the process of reliving past emotions. According to the authors, even biofeedback cannot produce such changes.

Evidence that whiplash can result in a somatoautonomic effect which causes subcortical EEG changes has been demonstrated by Liu et al. (58). In their study of 16 monkeys subject to whiplash (including control animals in which electrodes were implanted after whiplash), nearly all scalp, cortical, and subcortical EEG readings taken 6 to 8 weeks after the trauma were normal. Shortly thereafter, a hippocampal spiking developed which the authors categorized as a subclinical form of posttraumatic epilepsy

Somatoautonomic reflexes such as these are mediated by certain neural influences. Supraspinal excitation or inhibition apparently play an important role in determining the response of the various sympathetic preganglionic neurons (49). Many other neural influences involved in SAR are detailed in Chapter 8 Of course, the stimulus and the involved neuron are factors. For example, the segmental pathway is dominant in stimulating the smooth muscle of the gastrointestinal tract, and the suprasegmental pathway is more powerful in stimulating cardiac vascular and sudomotor neurons (49). Moreover, it has been concluded that localized stimuli evoke somatosympathetic reflexes which are mediated by spinal reflex pathways, but that in those reflexes in which a more generalized stimulus is involved, the supraspinal pathway is favored (49). These stimuli influence activity in the various levels of the neuroaxis, which in turn influences the sympathetic preganglionic neuron. Coote (49) has stated that such changes could well lead to altered autonomic motor responses.

Of course, such observations are not entirely new. MacKenzie (59) reported that physicians have frequently used counterirritation in the pit of the stomach to allay vomiting and that after operations involving the skin of the perineum, retention of urine follows. He identified these "effects of the stimulation of the skin on the viscera" in 1893, before the first chiropractic adjustment was given.

In light of the research reviewed in Chapters 8 and 13 as well as the studies reported in this chapter, it becomes apparent that the fixation hypothesis is a logical premise from which to build the SAR hypothesis. It is evident that this SAR hypothesis is based on a wealth of scientific study and observation; the degree of autonomic response that might be expected from the SF, however, cannot be determined at this time. If clinical research can continue to support the initial osteopathic clinical studies (40, 41, 60, 61), the SAR hypothesis would indeed appear to be the most logical justification for the use of chiropractic adjustment for conditions other than pain syndromes (3–6, 50, 62, 63).

Summary

Early osteopathic experimental observations demonstrated in the animal model that spinal lesions (spinal fixations, intervertebral subluxations) could cause circulatory changes that prompted alterations in gastric acidity, blood chemistry, and heart function among others (11-29). Chiropractors have suspected involvement of the somatoautonomic reflex (SAR) (2, 4, 7-9, 62), and current experimental findings suggest that this is a valid assumption (3, 6, 44, 45, 60, 61). This hypothesis, that spinal fixations could cause the somatic afferent bombardment of dorsal horn cells necessary to alter somatoautonomic reflexes or evoke abnormal autonomic reflexes, is termed the somatoautonomic reflex (SAR) hypothesis. It appears from medical and osteopathic clinical research that such reflexes can set into motion a wide variety of abnormal pathological and functional processes including such conditions as asthma, bronchitis, acute pulmonary atelectasis, muscular atrophy and degeneration, gastrointestinal complaints, coronary arteriospasm associated with ischemic heart disease, and pain actually referred to any portion of the body (10-29, 33-40). It is suggested that further clinical research on this mechanism is warranted and that the SAR hypothesis may be the most logical justification for the use of chiropractic adjustment for conditions other than pain syndromes (4-6, 50, 62, 63).

References

1. Korr IM (ed): *The Neurobiologic Mechanisms in Manipulative Therapy.* New York, Plenum, 1978, pp 91-127, 179-218.
2. Hviid H: A consideration of contemporary chiropractic theory. *J Nat Chiroprac Assoc* 25:17-18, 1955.
3. Korr IM: The spinal cord as organizer of disease processes: some preliminary perspectives. *J Am Osteopath Assoc* 76:89-99, 1976.
4. Haldeman S: Interactions between the somatic and visceral nervous systems. *ACA J Chiropractic* 5:57-64, 1971.
5. Haldeman S: Spinal and paraspinal receptors. *J Can Chiropractic Assoc* 17:28-32, 1972.
6. Denslow JS: The somatic component. *J Am Osteopath Assoc* 52:258-261, 1953.
7. Homewood AE: *The Neurodynamics of the Vertebral Subluxation.* Thornhill, Ontario, published privately, 1962.
8. Watkins RJ: Principles of nerve activity. Unpublished, 1978.
9. Verner JR: *The Science and Logic of Chiropractic.* Brooklyn, Cerasoli, 1941.
10. Burns L: Evidence of the existence of lesions. *Still Res Inst Bull* 5:14-15, 1917.
11. Deason J, Doron CL: Some immediate effects of bony lesions on vascular reflexes. *Still Res Inst Bull* 2:99-101, 1916.
12. Pengra CA, Alexander GA: Effects of spondylotherapic and osteopathic stimulation on the secretion of urine. *Still Res Inst Bull* 2:128-132, 1916.
13. Hoskins ER: A preliminary study of the motility of the gastro-intestinal tract in lesioned animals. *Still Res Inst Bull* 5:16-37, 1917.
14. Burns L: Changes in the gastric juice and the mucosa of guinea pigs with upper thoracic lesions. *Still Res Inst Bull* 7:27-36, 1931.
15. Burns L: Changes in the gastric juice and the stomach wall of guinea pigs with seventh and other lower thoracic lesion. *Still Res Inst Bull* 7:37-41, 1931.

16. Burns L: Immediate effects of certain manipulations upon the secretion of hydrochloric acid. *Still Res Inst Bull* 7:70–73, 1931.

17. Burns L: Acidity of the gastric juice in the progeny of lesioned rabbits. *Still Res Inst Bull* 7:79–98, 1931.

18. Burns L: Changes in the kidneys of guinea pigs with lesions of the twelfth and thirteenth thoracic vertebrae. *Still Res Inst Bull* 7:100–105, 1931.

19. Burns L: Changes in the kidneys and the urine due to the indirect effects of bony lesions. *Still Res Inst Bull* 7:121–124, 1931.

20. Burns L: Changes in tissue fluids due to vertebral lesions. *Still Res Inst Bull* 7:128–137, 1931.

21. Cherrill K, Whiting LD, Tweed L, Still CE: Costogenic anemia. *Still Res Inst Bull* 7:156–166, 1931.

22. Cherrill K, Whiting LD, Tweed L, Still CE: Pigments of the blood plasma. *Still Res Inst Bull* 7:174–179, 1931.

23. Tweed L: Physiology of the endocrines as affected by bony lesions. *Still Res Inst Bull* 7:167–173, 1931.

24. Burns L: *Growth Changes due to Vertebral Lesions.* Chicago, Still Research Institute, 1926.

25. Deason J: *On the Osteopathic Treatment of Diseases of the Ear, Nose and Throat.* Chicago, Still Research Institute, 1915.

26. Burns L, Chandler L, Rice R: *Pathogenesis of Visceral Disease following Vertebral Lesions.* Chicago, Still Research Institute, 1948, pp 193–211.

27. Bliss P: The vasomotor nerves of the lungs. *J Am Osteopath Assoc* 6:461–467, 1907.

28. Burns L: Viscero-somatic and somato-visceral spinal reflexes. *J Am Osteopath Assoc* 7:51–60, 1907.

29. Fichera AP, Celander DR: Effect of osteopathic manipulative therapy on autonomic tone as evidenced by blood pressure changes and activity of the fibrinolytic system. *J Am Osteopath Assoc* 68:72–74, 1969.

30. Kaliner M, Shelhamer JH, Davis PB, Smith LJ, Venter JC: Autonomic nervous system abnormalities and allergy. *Ann Intern Med* 96:349–357, 1982.

31. Ekman P, Levenson RW, Friesen WV: Autonomic nervous system activity distinguishes among emotions. *Science* 221:1208–1210, 1983.

32. Guyton AC: *Basic Human Physiology.* Philadelphia, Saunders, 1971, pp 297–298, 614–615.

33. Ussher NT: Spinal curvatures—visceral disturbances in relation thereto. *Calif West Med* 38:423–428, 1933.

34. Ussher NT: The viscerospinal syndrome—a new concept of visceromotor and sensory changes in relation to deranged spinal structures. *Ann Intern Med* 54:2057–2090, 1940.

35. Wills I, Atsatt RE: The viscerospinal syndrome: a confusing factor in surgical diagnosis. *Arch Surg* 29:661–668, 1934.

36. Murphy W, Wilson PT: A study of the value of osteopathic adjustment of the fourth and fifth thoracic vertebrae in a series of twenty cases of asthmatic bronchitis. *Boston Med Surg J* 192:440–442, 1925.

37. Pottenger FM: Important reflex relationships between the lungs and other viscera. *J Thorac Surg* 1.75–90, 1931.

38. Pottenger FM: The viscerospinal reflex. *Calif West Med* 38: June 1933.

39. Pottenger FM: *Symptoms of Visceral Disease.* St Louis. Mosby, 1953.

40. Rogers JT, Rogers JC: The role of osteopathic manipulative therapy in the treatment of coronary heart disease. *J Am Osteopath Assoc* 76:71–81, 1976.

41. Miller WD: Treatment of visceral disorders by manipulative therapy. In Goldstein M (ed): *The Research Status of Spinal Manipulative Therapy.* Washington, DC, Government Printing Office, 1975, pp 295–301.

152   THEORIES OF SUBLUXATION PATHOPHYSIOLOGY

42. DePace DM, Webber RH: Electrostimulation and morphologic study of the nerves to the bone marrow of the albino rat. *Acta Anat* 93:1–18, 1975.
43. Kuntz A, Richins C: Innervation of bone marrow. *J Comp Neurol* 83:213–222, 1945.
44. Sato A: The somatosympathetic reflexes: their physiological and clinical significance. In Goldstein M (ed): *The Research Status of Spinal Manipulative Therapy.* Washington, DC, Government Printing Office, 1975, pp 163–172.
45. Sato A, Schmidt RF: Somatosympathetic reflexes: afferent fibers, central pathways, discharge characteristics. *Phys Rev* 53:916–947, 1973.
46. Appenzeller O: Somatoautonomic reflexology—normal and abnormal. In Korr IM (ed): *The Neurobiologic Mechanisms in Manipulative Therapy.* New York, Plenum, 1978, pp 179–217.
47. Kiyomi, K: Autonomic system reactions caused by excitation of somatic afferents: study of cutaneo-intestinal reflex. In Korr IM (ed): *The Neurobiologic Mechanisms in Manipulative Therapy.* New York, Plenum, 1978, pp 219–227.
48. Kuntz A, Haselwood LA: Circulatory reactions in the gastrointestinal tract elicited by localized cutaneous stimulation. *Am Heart J* 20:743–749, 1940.
49. Coote JH: Somatic sources of afferent input as factors in aberrant autonomic, sensory and motor function. In Korr IM (ed): *The Neurobiologic Mechanisms in Manipulative Therapy.* New York, Plenum, 1978, pp 91–127.
50. Korr IM: Sustained sympathicotonia as a factor in disease. In Korr IM (ed): *The Neurobiologic Mechanisms in Manipulative Therapy.* New York, Plenum, 1978, pp 229–268.
51. Norman J, Whitwam JG: The vagal contribution to changes in heart rate evoked by stimulation of cutaneous nerves in the dog. *J Physiol* 234:89P–90P, 1973.
52. Matoba T, Ohkita Y, Chiba M, Toshima H: Noninvasive assessment of the autonomic nervous tone in angina pectoris: an application of digital plethysmography with auditory stimuli. *Angiology* 34:127–136, 1983.
53. Schraeder PL, Lathers CM: Cardiac neural discharge and epileptogenic activity in the cat: an animal model for unexplained death. *Life Sci* 32:1371–1382, 1983.
54. Gutstein WH, LaTaillade JN, Lewis L: Role of vasoconstriction in experimental arteriosclerosis. *Circ Res* 10:925–932, 1962.
55. Gutstein WH, Harrison J, Parl F, Kiu G, Avitable M: Neural factors contribute to atherogenesis. *Science* 199:449–451, 1978.
56. Droste PL, Beckman DL: Pulmonary effects of prolonged sympathetic stimulation. *Proc Soc Exp Biol Med* 146:352–353, 1974.
57. Editors: Autonomic abnormalities in asthma. *Lancet* 1:1224–1225, 1982.
58. Liu YK, Chandran KB, Heath RG, Unterharnscheidt F: Subcortical EEG changes in rhesus monkeys following experimental hyperextension-hyperflexion (whiplash). *Spine* 9:329–338, 1984.
59. MacKenzie J: Some points bearing on the association of sensory disorders and visceral disease. *Brain* 16:321–354, 1893.
60. Denslow JS, Hassett CC: The central excitatory state associated with postural abnormalities. *J Neurophysiol* 5:393–402, 1942.
61. Denslow JS: An analysis of the variability of spinal reflex thresholds. *J Neurophysiol* 7:207–215, 1944.
62. Haldeman S: The clinical basis for discussion of mechanisms in manipulative therapy. In Korr IM (ed): *The Neurobiologic Mechanisms in Manipulative Therapy.* New York, Plenum, 1978, pp 53–75.
63. Korr IM: Proprioceptors and the behavior of lesioned segments. In Stark EH (ed): *Osteopathic Medicine.* Acton, MA, Publication Sciences Group, 1975, pp 183–199.

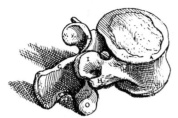

Chapter 12

Neurodystrophic Hypothesis

*C*hiropractic was founded on the idea of body tone; thus, Palmer (1) writes:

> The amount of nerve tension determines health or disease. In health there is normal tension, known as tone, the normal activity, strength and excitability of the various organs and functions as observed in a state of health. The kind of disease depends upon what nerves are too tense or too slack.

This idea of body tone has been determined to be sheer quackery by more than a majority of medical investigators throughout this century and for plausible reasons (2–4). Medical researchers have sought and succeeded in determining the causative agents in many diseases, most of which responded well to antibiotic and other therapies (5). Moreover, North American immunologists have succeeded in determining that a variety of factors (including genetic, cell-mediated, lymphoid, thymic, and hormonal) appear to play roles in the defense of the human body to disease (6–24).

Immunologists have succeeded in demonstrating specific primary and secondary responses to antigens *in vitro* and ways to inhibit such responses *in vitro* (5–9). The results of immunizing the peoples of the world to a number of diseases have been mixed, however (25–33). Although smallpox has apparently been wiped out, other less encouraging mass immunization programs such as for the supposed "swine flu" epidemic in 1976 have met with disaster, have cost lives, and have wasted millions of dollars in the process (29, 33). Nevertheless, according to much of the literature, there appears to be little reason for immunologists, medical doctors, scientists, or anyone else to believe in the chiropractic tenet that intervertebral subluxations can play a role in the genesis of organic disease.

Since the first edition of this text, psychoneuroimmunology has developed as an emerging field of scientific study. A theme that is central to much of the research from this field is that there is interaction between central nervous system function and immunity (34–41). This research, of course, contradicts traditional medical and scientific thought that there was no relationship between the nervous system and immunity and, therefore, chiropractic manipulation could have no effect on immune function (3, 4). These researchers and previous investigators in the U.S.S.R., Germany, and North America have made discoveries that appear to substantiate the chiropractic *neurodystrophic* hypothesis (42–66). This hypothesis is that neural dysfunction is stressful to the visceral and other body structures and that this "lowered tissue resistance" can modify the nonspecific and specific immune responses and alter the trophic function of the involved nerves (1, 67–74). Some of these researchers (39–41, 56–66, 75–86) have concluded that the nervous system is intimately involved in specific and nonspecific body defenses. For instance, the classic works of Selye (42, 43) and others (49–51) in North America have recently demonstrated neuroendocrine-immune connections in experiments and clinical investigations. Moreover, psychoneuroimmunologists have now documented a connection between immunologic competence and the anterior hypothalamus (36–38, 44–48). The major emphasis of this chapter is on clarification of these mechanisms and on providing an answer to the question, "What role does the nervous system play in specific and nonspecific body defenses?"

Known Factors in the Immune Respose

According to current North American immunological concepts, the specific immune response in humans appears to be based on the classical precipitin reaction (5–9). Hence, when an antigen (Ag) (viz., any foreign substance capable of eliciting an antibody response) solution is mixed with its corresponding antisera (i.e., containing antibodies specific for the administered Ag) *in vitro*, a precipitate is formed. The reaction depends on the valency of the antigen, which varies according to the size and the species synthesizing the antibody. Included among the factors regulating the binding of antigen to antibody are the normal intermolecular forces that regulate binding between any two unrelated proteins (i.e., *coulombic* or the attraction between oppositely charged ionic groups; *hydrogen bonding; hydrophobic bonding*; and *Van der Waals'* bonding, or the interaction between the external "electron clouds"). Antibodies that when combined with antigen react to form a precipitate are known as *precipitins*. What is important, however, is that the actual attraction of antibody to antigen is thought to be totally independent of direct neural regulation. In thousands of experiments, immunologists have thus succeeded in showing that the primary and secondary immune responses can not only be demonstrated *in vitro* but can also be inhibited *in vitro* (5–9).

Experiments on rats and guinea pigs have demonstrated that the actual "memory" for any given antigen is coded into the DNA of small lymphocytes, as well as macrophages; again the nervous system is not directly involved (5–7, 10). Hence, in one series of experiments (5), immunologists injected specific antigens into "virgin" rats (animals that had not been previously exposed to any specific antigen). The animals—having thus been primed—were then operated on, and small lymphocytes from these animals were transferred into other unprimed genetically identical recipients by injection. Injection of the antigen into the unprimed animals produced strong secondary antibody responses. Hence, the small lymphocytes carried the "sensitization" to the antigen from the first to the second group of animals, which is proof positive that the actual memory for the secondary antibody response was coded into the small lymphocytes (6).

Further experiments have demonstrated that two types of lymphocytes (viz., "bursa equivalent" or *B cells*, which are thymus independent, and thymus-dependent or *T cells*) appear to work in cooperation with macrophages to stimulate antibody synthesis (5–7, 14–23). One current model that is based on *The Clonal Selection Theory of Acquired Immunity* of Burnet (11) holds that when antigen is present inside the body, the T cell lymphocytes adhere simultaneously to macrophages and to the antigen (Figure 12.1). This linkage stimulates the T cells to send basically three "messages." One message occurs when the T cell releases "receptor" protein molecules, which have been coded for the antigen, throughout the area of invasion. When monocytes pick up these proteins, they immediately are activated to become aggressive

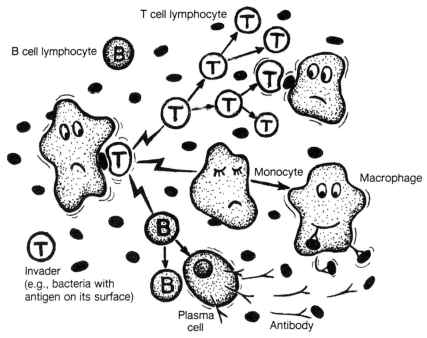

Figure 12.1. One well-known model of antigen-antibody interaction holds that adherence of T cell lymphocytes to antigen and macrophage triggers a threefold T cell response: a) call for increased T cell production; b) cause monocytes to become active macrophages; and c) call for B cells to proliferate and become plasma cells that synthesize antibodies. Antibodies are Y-shaped proteins that latch onto antigens on invading bacteria, etc. The shaft of the antibody, in turn, attaches to macrophages which may then more quickly engulf and destroy the invader. (Adapted from Gore R: The awesome worlds within a cell. *Natl Geographic* 150:355–395, 1976.)

macrophages. Other "messages" go out to produce more T cells and to signal B cells to proliferate and become plasma cells (which in turn produce and release antibodies specific for the invading antigen). Much evidence supports this and similar models based on Burnet's theory, which is undoubtedly the most widely accepted theory of immunity in North America today (5–7, 14–23).

Immunologists have performed a wide variety of experiments that indicate that other factors may play important roles in the immune response. Factors that have been positively identified as modifying and at least partially controlling the specific as well as the nonspecific immune response to disease include cell-mediated, humoral, lymphoid, thymic, genetic, nutritional, endocrine, neural, and stress-related factors. The latter three are discussed in detail in the next few sections, as they are probably the most important chiropractically.

Cell-mediated immunity (CMI) plays a prominent role in protecting the body from a variety of pathogens. In a classic series of experiments, immunologists have shown that certain organisms may not respond to an attack when antibodies are the lone defenders but will readily succumb when lymphocytes are actively involved (6). This was shown by injecting donor rats with moderate doses of *Mycobacterium tuberculosis*. The animals overcame this infection and became immune to further injections. Later injections into these animals sensitized to *M. tuberculosis* resulted in vigorous secondary immune responses. Amazingly, if another different organism (e.g., *Listeria monocytogenes*) simultaneously is injected during a second challenge with *M. tuberculosis*, the animals respond by killing both invaders (when normally the *Listeria* infection alone would overcome the animals). These experiments suggested that the initiation of a specific secondary immune response enhanced a simultaneous nonspecific response to other unrelated organisms with similar growth habits (i.e., both *Listeria* and the tubercle bacilli may live and grow inside macrophages, even following ingestion by phagocytosis).

Further experiments showed that this nonspecific response was cell-mediated by T cell lymphocytes. This was demonstrated by first infecting a series of rats with *M. tuberculosis*. From these initial donor rats, specific immune sera, macrophages, and lymphocytes were taken and independently injected into three other groups of rats. Rats that received only the specific immune sera (containing specific antibodies for *M. tuberculosis*) were challenged with injections of *L. monocytogenes* and *M. tuberculosis*. They became infected. A second group of rats received macrophages from the donor rats; following injection with *L. monocytogenes* and *M. tuberculosis*, they too became infected. The third group of rats received lymphocytes from the donor animals, however, and became immune to further challenge with both *Listeria* and the tubercle bacilli (6) (Figure 12.2). Recent experimentation has conclusively documented these findings and has suggested that in human leprosy, CMI as opposed to humoral immunity (viz., specific immune sera, specific antibody response) is crucial to the control of the disease (6). Other bacteria and

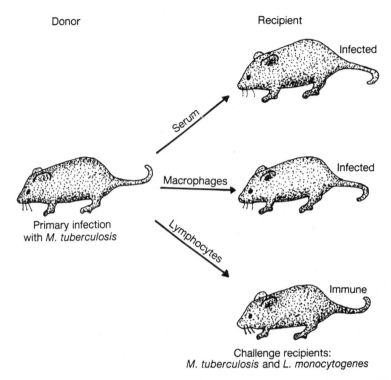

Figure 12.2.   After injection of rats with immune sera, macrophages, and lymphocytes from rats infected with *M. tuberculosis,* only the animals receiving lymphocytes are immune to further challenge by *L. monocytogenes* and *M. tuberculosis*. (Adapted from Roitt IM: *Essential Immunology.* London, Blackwell Scientific Publications, 1974, p 166.)

viruses have been similarly shown to be overcome by cell-mediated rather than humoral immunity. (Note that lymphocytes are considered part of both humoral and cell-mediated responses to disease.)

Humoral immunity is, of course, fundamental to any specific defense response to bacteria, viruses, protozoa and, possibly, helminths (5–7). The immunoglobulins function as the specific antibodies that fight antigens that enter the body (i.e., the humoral response). The previously mentioned precipitin reaction (considered a classic humoral response) is used primarily by immunologists who wish to determine the antibody content of the immune serum or the valency of the antigen.

The thymus gland has been implicated in aging and in the immune response (5–7, 12, 49, 50). The latter is due to the now-established fact that T cells must pass through or be acted on by this gland before they are activated, to participate properly in the immune response. Since T cells are central to the clonal selection model mentioned previously, it is easy to see that the thymus is now viewed as a primary organ of immunity. Many experiments have shown that the thymus is crucial to the immune response. Two classic experiments, however, have principally documented the thymic role in immunologic competence. In one study, thymectomy of mice at birth resulted in decreased circulating lymphocyte counts, impairment of graft rejection, decreased normal humoral antibody response to many antigens, and general wasting due to the inability of the mice to fight infections (6). In the other study, adult mice were irradiated to destroy their immunological competence. One subgroup of irradiated mice were then given injections of bone marrow cells, whereas the other subgroup of irradiated mice were given injections of adult spleen and adult lymph node cells. Injections of bone marrow cells were not effective in restoring immunological competence to previously irradiated mice. Immunological competence was restored, however, in the groups of irradiated mice receiving injections of adult spleen and adult lymph node cells (6). These and other authors concluded that the thymus acts on blood marrow cells to make them immunologically competent (5–7, 12, 49, 50). Although it was once thought that thymus gland activity was independent of neural regulation, there is now evidence that the CNS is a regulator of thymic activity (87).

It has long been known that genetic factors are fundamental to the immune response. It has been shown not only that the resistance of different species is highly variable but also that the actual memory for the secondary response is coded into at least the DNA of T cell lymphocytes and probably of macrophages (as previously mentioned in this section) (5–7, 10). Chandra (13) has recently shown that malnutrition in young rats not only can greatly impair their immune response (by causing reduced growth, involution of lymphoid organs, and lymphopenia) but also can impair antibody formation in the next two generations of animals (i.e., their progeny). These findings were compared with clinical findings, and it was suggested that impaired immunocompetence following intrauterine malnutrition may endure for a long time. It was further suggested that immunodeficiency diseases such as autoimmunity, neoplasias, and frequent infections may appear in the human mother as well as in her offspring as a result of this malnutrition. It was thus shown that malnutrition may interfere with the immune response and that the effects are passed down to future generations apparently by genetic code (13).

In addition to cell-mediated, humoral, lymphoid, thymic, genetic, and nutritional factors affecting or participating in the immune response which appear to be independent of neural influence, there are other factors that would appear to lend credibility to the neurodystrophic hypothesis.

Concept of Stress

The classic works of Selye (42, 43), which summarized thousands of studies by other scientists, demonstrated for the first time that exposure to stress can cause "diseases of adaptation." Selye ultimately was credited with defining and revising the theories surrounding stress into one comprehensive model which has since been praised around the world. The "general adaptation syndrome" (GAS) is a model for stress capable of explaining the many and diverse physiological reactions to various stressors. The GAS begins with the "alarm reaction" (AR). When the human organism first is exposed to stress (either a *systemic* stressor or a *topical* stressor), the AR begins which may include any or all of the following:

1. Adrenocortical enlargement with histologic signs of hyperactivity. This systemic nonspecific reaction includes secretion of increased amounts of cortisone and adrenocorticotropic hormone (ACTH).
2. Thymicolymphatic involution including eosinopenia, lymphopenia, and polynucleosis.
3. Gastrointestinal tract ulcers.
4. Miscellaneous signs of damage or shock.

Following the initial response of AR, the human physiological response shifts to one of resistance or the "stage of resistance" (SR).

The SR will be functional as long as the endocrine and other systems are capable of responding normally. Various "conditioning factors" are able to modify the hormonal actions and hence the SR, however. Such "conditioning factors" include the following:

1. Hereditary, nutritional, and age factors.
2. Increased protein diet results in increased production of corticotrophic hormone.
3. Increased sodium ion concentration augments the action of mineralocorticoids (MCs).
4. Stress itself is probably the most effective and common factor in conditioning the actions of adaptive hormones. Thus *systemic* stressors (which stimulate the GAS response) increase the antiphlogistic, lympholytic, catabolic, and hyperglycemic actions of antiphlogistic corticoids (ACs), while *topical* stressors increase the salient effects of adaptive hormones. Topical stressors modify the course of inflammation by eliciting a phlogistic response which actually facilitates inflammation. A topical stressor stimulates a local adaptation syndrome (LAS) response.

These conditioning factors determine whether the stress will be manifest by the so-called diseases of adaptation (including such experimentally and clinically verified diseases as hypertensive and inflammatory rheumatic diseases, nephrosis, nephritis, nephrosclerosis, hypertension, vascular lesions, rheumatic fever, rheumatoid arthritis, gastrointestinal ulcers, aldosteronism, periarteritis nodosa, hyperthyroidism, thyroiditis, certain types of liver disease, Von Gierke's disease, and certain tumors) or by the "physiologic adaptation syndrome" which is the response that allows our bodies to adapt to stress rather than to succumb to it (Figure 12.3). In addition to the aforementioned conditioning factors, events that will inhibit the GAS and may result in a disease (or diseases) of adaptation include the following:

1. Any absolute increase or decrease in the amount of adaptive hormones (e.g., corticoids, ACTH, somatotropic hormone (STH), and aldosterone) that are produced during stress.
2. Any absolute increase or decrease in the amount of adaptive hormones that become retained in their respective peripheral target organs during stress.
3. Any disproportion in the relative secretion of various antag-

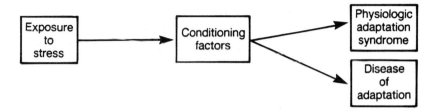

Figure 12.3. According to the Selye (42, 43) model, the stage of resistance will be functional unless it is modified by the various conditioning factors, which may result in physiologic adaptation or disease of adaptation.

onistic adaptive hormones (the actions of ACTH and other ACs are antagonistic to the actions of STH and the prophlogistic corticoids or PCs) during stress.

4. The production of metabolic derangements that alter the target organ's normal response to adaptive hormones. Stress can produce such metabolic derangements through the previously mentioned "conditioning factors."

5. Any abnormal neural, renal, hepatic, and/or other responses.

The entire GAS is therefore based on the idea that under optimum conditions the body is capable of responding to various stressors by adapting to them. When the hypophyseoadrenocortical system is not functioning correctly, however, there is a relative increase in the pathogenicity of many systemic and local stressor agents. It is thus easy to see why diseases caused by inability of the body to adapt to stressors are termed diseases of adaptation. Other body systems are involved, obviously, in the process of adaptation. Hence, according to researchers, an abnormal response by the nervous system—or of other major body systems—may play an important role in the etiology of diseases of adaptation.

Selye (42, 43) and these investigators determined that the nervous system is involved in the hypophyseoadrenocortical response to stress by a number of pathways. Frustration, for example, may act as a neurogenic stressor to stimulate great increases in ACTH secretions. By experiments with animals it was shown that such a "neurogenic stressor" follows a path through the hypothalamus to the anterior lobe of the pituitary (adenohypophysis) where ACTH is secreted into the systemic circulation. By another pathway it was found that autonomic nervous system stimuli causing vasoconstriction actually prepare the tissues of the body (extrarenal) for the antiphlogistic effects of cortisol and cortisone. Further connections between the neuroendocrine systems also were demonstrated. Thus, the hypophyseoadrenocortical system was shown to affect the central nervous system (e.g., corticoids may cause anesthesia, euphoria, depression, and even transient paralysis).

These findings, which are based on more than 30,000 scientific studies, obviously have become extremely important to the chiropractic profession. For the first time ever, pathways (Figure 12.4) have been scientifically demonstrated which verified that the nervous system participates in the response to stress and may therefore be a factor in any of the so-called diseases of adaptation.

Neuroendocrine-Immune Connection

The studies of Selye (42, 43) demonstrated for the first time that the response to stress was coordinated by a neuroendocrine mechanism. Yet during the 1950s, there was little evidence from the North American literature to demonstrate any connections between this neuroendocrine response and immunologic competence. Denckla (50) and others (47–49, 51–53) recently have shown that there is such a connection.

At the Harvard Medical School, Denckla (50) thoroughly reviewed the literature and noted various interactions between age and the neuroendocrine and immune systems. Through various studies it was shown that the pituitary was connected with the immune system; two hormones controlled by the pituitary— growth hormone and thyroid-stimulating hormone—were shown to be beneficial to immunologic competence. Xenograft rejection (viz., a rejection of a graft of tissue transplanted from another species of animal) is considered a valid monitor of immune system competence. In one series of experiments by Bilder and Denckla (51), it was shown that xenograft rejection in young and old intact rats took place in 6.0 and 13.8 days, respectively. After removal of the pituitary gland and later injection of thyroxine (T_4) and growth hormone, however, the older (64 weeks) rats rejected xenografts in approximately 6.5 days, a rejection time that was not significantly different from that for younger (4 weeks) rats. This dem-

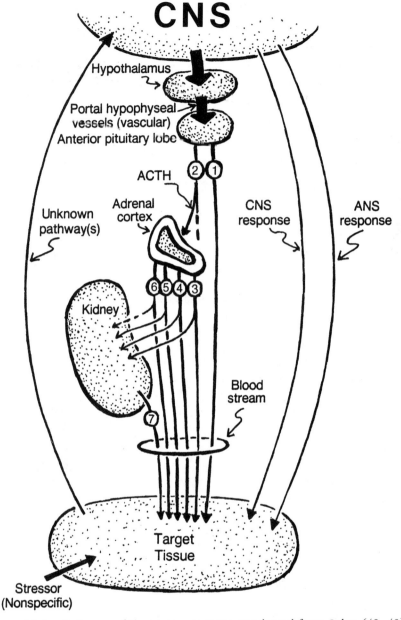

Figure 12.4. Pathways of the stress response as adapted from Selye (42, 43) illustrate that the CNS is an important mediator of stress in humans. Endocrine glands secrete the following hormones needed for this response: *1*) somatotropic hormone (STH), *2*) adrenocorticotropic hormone (ACTH), *3*) prophlogistic corticoid, *4*) noradrenalin, *5*) adrenalin, *6*) antiphlogistic corticoid, and *7*) renal pressor substance. In some cases, according to Selye, the unknown pathways that alert the CNS to the presence of a nonspecific stressor could be the nervous impulse (0)

onstrated that the pituitary was a significant factor in certain aspects of maturation and senescence within the immune system. It was shown by these researchers and others that the decline in sensitivity of target tissues to pituitary hormones (as measured by minimal O_2 consumption) with age was not due to a decrease in hormonal levels. It was suggested, instead, that with advancing age the pituitary releases a factor that is increasingly detrimental to the immune response (51). Physiologists have determined that pituitary secretions are under the influence of humoral and neural influences; hence, there are now data that implicate connections between the neuroendocrine system and aging of certain components of the immune system (49–51).

Selye may have opened the door to neuroendocrine and/or stress research, but psychiatrists in the mid-1970s appear to have walked through that door. Stein et al. (44) reviewed the literature, including their own studies, that had convincingly demonstrated psychosocial and neural influences on the immune system. In their experiments, the central nervous system and, specifically, the hypothalamus were demonstrated to have direct effects on the humoral immune response (see also "Anterior Hypothalamus and Immunologic Competence" in this chapter) (44, 45). Hence, in various experimental studies in mice, it has been shown that psychosocial factors can modify host resistance to infection with herpes simplex virus, poliomyelitis virus, coxsackie B virus, polyoma virus, and vesicular stomatitis virus. Clinical findings have verified these observations, according to the authors. Other psychosocial factors increased the susceptibility of these animals to infection by other agents but were not factors that necessarily involved the nervous system; in contrast, the previous named agents all increased in relative pathogenicity when psychological stressors mediated through the nervous system were applied to the test animals. Even more astonishing were the findings that psychosocial factors, again mediated through the nervous system, were conclusively shown to affect the development, course, and outcome of neoplastic disorders (44). In their review of literature they cited studies that showed that infantile stimulation affects the development, course, and outcome of cancer (Walker 256 sarcoma) injected into rats. In mice, the survival time after transplantation with lymphoid leukemia was significantly decreased with previous infantile stimulation. Mammary carcinomas and survival time following various subcellular injections in experimental animals also were modified by psychosocial factors mediated through the nervous system (44).

Research along similar lines by Monjan and Collector (54) has demonstrated not only that stress in clinical animals sometimes can depress immune responsiveness but also that other environmental stressors may enhance immune responsiveness.

Murphy et al. (55) have shown that hippocampal lesions promote increased plasma corticosterone levels, as well as gastric ulcers, in animals confronted with stress. When various groups of rats were restrained (a psychological stress), all animals with hippocampal lesions developed ulcers in the glandular portion of the stomach (mean total length of ulcer was 3.78 mm). Only one animal in the cortical control group (viz., animals with that portion of the cortex above the hippocampus removed bilaterally by aspiration) developed an ulcer (length, 0.50 mm). Only two animals in the normal group developed ulcers with simple restraint (mean total length of ulcer was 0.37 mm). Among animals stressed by simple restraint, it was found that those with hippocampal lesions had significantly more ulceration ($p = 0.001$) than did control animals (55).

Riley (41), after research and an extensive literature review, has concluded that animal housing, unnecessary handling of laboratory rats and animals, and other variables may be responsible for the often-conflicting research regarding stress and the immune system. He distinguishes between direct stress-induced pathologies and stress-induced modulation of immune responsiveness. Hence, with acute or chronic stress an incipient or latent neoplasm or infection that is either preexistent or is introduced during the stress state can be induced into an overt pathology. Likewise, viral and neoplastic pathologies that are under partial or complete control by cell-mediated immunological defenses may be clearly enhanced by stress. In the case of neoplastic pathologies, the enhancing effects of stress on disease occur as a result of the adverse effects of stress on specific immunological elements of the host, which suggests an indirect role of stress on pathology. Riley (41) suggested the following:

1. If there is no underlying disease, stress-associated infectious or neoplastic pathologies will not be observed.

2. The effects of stress will not be observed even if there are latent pathologies, unless the unimpaired immunological system is in partial or complete control of the disease.
3. The adverse effects of stress will be observed only when the host immune defenses and the resident pathology are in a state of equilibrium, which thus permits stress to modify and impair the host's immunological competence.

That stress can impair immunity in direct proportion to the intensity of the stressor was documented recently by Keller et al. (38). Measuring the number of circulating lymphocytes by phytohemagglutinin stimulation of lymphocytes in whole blood and isolated cultures, these scientists found that a series of graded stresses (home cage controls, apparatus controls restrained by tape and electrodes attached but with no current delivered, and low- and high-shock animals) progressively suppressed lymphocytic function (38).

In an extensive review of recent human studies regarding the relationship of stress to immune function, Locke (39) has identified three important factors: duration and proximity of the stressor, adaptive capacity of the individual, and differential effects of various stressors on various immunologic components.

It appears that a wide variety of psychosocial factors, when mediated through the central nervous system, are able to decrease the level of immunologic competence and increase the relative pathogenicity of infectious agents and neoplastic disorders (44–54).

Reflex Mechanism of Immunologic Competence

While Selye and his many colleagues were documenting the role of the nervous system in the response to stress throughout the 1950s, other researchers in the U.S.S.R., Germany, and North America were finding evidence that appears to conflict with the previously mentioned model of antigen-antibody interaction. Several of these investigators who utilized radioactive isotopes in classic pulse-chase experiments appear to have demonstrated that antibody formation may be initiated by some nervous system reflex.

Speransky (56, 57) performed a series of experiments at the

All-Union Institute of Experimental Medicine in Leningrad throughout the 1920s and the 1930s. In early experimentation on epilepsy, Speransky found that introduction of any of a variety of substances into the nervous system resulted in epileptic attacks. Neither the substance nor the nerve were found to vary the course of the disease. Moreover, intravenous injection of the same substances (croton oil, phenol, formalin, acids, bile, etc.) into the blood was not accompanied by the development of convulsive attacks. In this way it was shown that epilepsy was of reflex origin. Speransky's research thus began by study of the role of the nervous system in various disease processes but progressed quickly. It had previously been known that tetanus toxoid could be injected into the leg of a dog and that antitoxin introduced into the sciatic nerve of the same animal would act as a chemical barrier, blockading passage of the tetanus antigen. In one classic series of experiments, Speransky injected normal serum into the sciatic nerve to achieve the same blockade against the tetanus antigen. Incredibly, Speransky found that even injection of tetanus toxoid into the nerve would blockade passage of the previous tetanus toxoid inoculation. In fact, in some cases, tetanus toxoid acted as a more efficient barrier than tetanus antitoxin (when injected into canine sciatic nerve to blockade intramuscular injection of tetanus toxoid). Further experimentation with other diseases and animals led Speransky and his associates to the ultimate conclusion that the nervous system reacted to various noxious stimuli in a more direct way than had ever previously been suspected (56):

> The appraisal of these data led so often to a conflict with the many existing views that very soon we perceived the necessity of giving up the study of isolated questions. By the force of circumstances, we were compelled to pass to a revision of the conceptions of the basic processes of general physiology, from the point of view of the nervous component in their origin and history.

Discoveries made by Speransky were not totally unique. In North America, Kuntz (58–60) reviewed the literature including many studies recorded in German and found studies by Reitler (1924), Bogendorfer (1927, 1932), Belak (1939), Illenyi and Borzsak (1938), Frei (1939), and Hoff (1942) that appeared to substantiate a role for the nervous system in regulating immune reactions. For example, in the study by Reitler, according to Kuntz, antibody formation was initiated in rabbits by injection of antigen into an ear following ligation of its vessels. The ear was amputated within 3 seconds of antigenic injection. Thus it was demonstrated that antibody titer increased reflexly and in the absence of antigen in the circulating blood.

According to Kuntz (60), the data showed "that the production of immune substances represents specific reflex secretory reactions to specific stimuli. . . . [and] that an immune reaction once initiated may continue in the absence of nervous influences." It should be noted, however, that several important questions were raised by this experiment, which had been previously performed by Speransky (56) and others (77) with similar results. It was suggested by other scientists that perhaps the antigen, even in that short amount of time, had been able to diffuse into the proximal tissues and hence into the systemic circulation (77). It was also suggested that perhaps the operation was not sterile. If this were true, substances other than antigen could have stimulated a polyclonal response (a nonspecific increase in antibody). It was pointed out to this author by an immunologist at a major medical school that an endotoxin, lipopolysaccharide, or a gram-negative microorganism could stimulate such a response, which would thereby invalidate the study.

Although because of these and similar criticisms of this initial research most North American scientists (notable exceptions included Kuntz and Selye) did not accept the conclusions, others in Russia began an active review of these data. From preliminary studies by Gordienko et al. (61) at the Rostov-on-Don State Medical Institute, it was concluded that the reflex theory of antibody formation proposed by Speransky, Reitler, Freidberger, and others was credible.

Because of the success of their preliminary studies, Gordienko et al. decided to determine more accurately the possibility of reflex antibody formation. Thus, they performed 98 experiments on rabbits divided into three groups (62) (Figure 12.5). In order to determine the rate of absorption of antigen, Group 1 rabbits were injected with the highly radioactive phosphorus isotope (^{32}P). A vaccine containing 800 million to 1 billion microorganisms was injected intracutaneously into the tip of the other ear in Group 1 animals and in Group 2 (control) animals. Since antigen used in this experiment was in the form of a colloidal

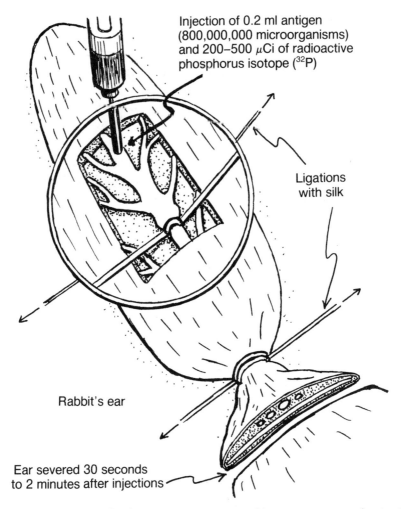

Injection of 0.2 ml antigen
(800,000,000 microorganisms)
and 200–500 μCi of radioactive
phosphorus isotope (^{32}P)

Ligations
with silk

Rabbit's ear

Ear severed 30 seconds
to 2 minutes after injections

Figure 12.5. In Gordienko's experiments on rabbits, one group of animals received injection of radioactive isotope ^{32}P), as well as injection of 800 million microorganisms in typhoid vaccine solution. The absence of the isotope in carotid artery following severance of the ear and the increase in agglutinin titer taken 7 days later strongly implied a neural reflex involvement in immunity.

suspension, it was said to have been absorbed into the tissues at a rate slower than that of the radioactive phosphorus isotope. The phosphorus was injected into the auricular nerve at the distal end of the rabbit's ear (the auricular nerve had been isolated, raised, and ligated). The entire ear was tightly constricted at its base with a silken ligature. In this series, as well as in all of Gordienko's experiments in which ^{32}P was utilized, massive amounts of radio-active phosphorus isotope were injected into the nerve (200 to 500 μCi). Two minutes following injection of ^{32}P and antigen, the ear was severed at its base. Cessation of absorption of ^{32}P was determined by noting changes in blood radioactivity (carotid artery) both before the introduction of radioactive phosphorus isotope and immediately following to several minutes following section of the ear. Agglutinin titers before and 7 days after the injection were compared. Results of this experiment (Table 12.1) showed that the variations in blood radioactivity (following intro-duction of phosphorus isotope into rabbit ear ligated at its root and later sectioned) are negligible and fall within normal limits. These researchers concluded that ligation of the ear with silken ligature guarantees negligible or minimal (less than 10,000 micro-organisms/kg animal weight) absorption of antigen introduced into the skin distal to the base, when the ear is severed at its base within 2 minutes. They estimated that total antigen resorption under such conditions could not exceed 1% or 2%. Yet analysis of agglutinin titers (Table 12.2) showed significant increases in 12 of 15 animals (62). Such increases could not be explained by accidental resorption of small amounts (under 10,000 microorga-nisms/kg animal weight) of antigen, since according to Gordienko et al. (62) other researchers had previously demonstrated that at

Table 12.1.   Carotid artery radioactivity before and after ^{32}P injection into ligated and severed rabbit ear[a]

Rabbit no.	^{32}P introduced (μCi)	Impulses/min/ml blood before introduction of ^{32}P	Cpm/ml blood immediately after introduction of ^{32}P and severance of ear
2	200	39–41	37–44
3	180	32–35	35–37
4	200	32–35	32–35
5	200	40–42	38–43
6	200	36–40	36–41
7	200	35–35	45–45
8	200	38–42	38–45
9	200	40–41	40–44

[a] From Gordienko AN, Kiseleva VI, Saakov BA, Bondarev IM, Zhigalini LI: The possibility of a reflex mechanism producing antibodies when antigen acts on skin receptors. In Gordienko AN (ed): *Control of Immunogenesis by the Nervous System.* Washington, DC, National Technical Information Service, 1958, pp 44–52 (62).

Table 12.2.   Agglutinin titers to typhoid vaccine before and after severance of rabbit ear[a]

Rabbit no.	Initial agglutinin titer	Agglutinin titer after 7 days
2	1:20	1:160
3	1:80	1:320
4	1:20	1:80
5	1.10	1:80
6	1:20	1:80
7	1:10	1:160
8	1:40	1:160
9	1:40	1:160
457	1:00	1:40
430	1:00	1:00
644	1:00	1:00
235	1:00	1:640
213	1:00	1:00
230	1:00	1:2560
151	1:00	1:1280

[a] From Gordienko AN, Kiseleva VI, Saakov BA, Bondarev IM, Zhigalini LI: The possibility of a reflex mechanism producing antibodies when antigen acts on skin receptors. In Gordienko AN (ed): *Control of Immunogenesis by the Nervous System.* Washington, DC, National Technical Information Service 1958, pp 44–52 (62).

least 100,000 microorganisms/kg animal weight must enter the blood before agglutinin titers rise to the levels shown in these experiments.

To establish that the reaction of the agglutinin titer was specific (not simply a polyclonal response, etc.), these researchers duplicated this experiment in another series of rabbits (Group 3) with use of paratyphoid B vaccine; as a control, agglutinin titers were made of paratyphoid A vaccine which was not injected. Had the agglutinin responses previously seen been due to some polyclonal response from infection of the rabbit ears, agglutinin titers to both paratyphoid B and paratyphoid A would be expected to rise. Data showed, however, that the reaction was specific only for the paratyphoid B antigen that had been introduced into the rabbit ear (62) (Table 12.3).

In another series of experiments, Gordienko et al. (63) determined that when various antigens contact nervous system receptors in the skin and blood vessels, specific bioelectric potentials are created that vary according to the antigen. These changes in the normal neural discharge were monitored electrophysiologically (Table 12.4). Control animals were given injections of phys-

Table 12.3. Alterations in agglutinin titers before and after injection of paratyphoid B vaccine and subsequent severance of rabbit ear with antigen depot[a]

Rabbit no.	Initial titer Paratyphoid		Titer after 7 days Paratyphoid	
	A	B	A	B
46	0	0	0	640
449	0	0	20	320
485	0	0	0	320
464	0	0	0	20
524	0	0	0	80
547	0	0	20	20
663	0	20	20	0
479	0	0	20	80
240	0	0		0
336	20	20	20	80

[a] From Gordienko AN, Kiseleva VI, Saakov BA, Bondarev IM, Zhigalini LI: The possibility of a reflex mechanism producing antibodies when antigen acts on skin receptors. In Gordienko AN (ed): *Control of Immunogenesis by the Nervous System.* Washington, DC, National Technical Information Service, 1958, pp 44–52 (62).

Table 12.4. Effects of various antigens and control solution on amplitude and velocity of nerve conduction (auricular and lateral femoral cutaneous nerves)[a]

Antigen[b]	Conduction velocity (oscillations/sec)	Amplitude (μV)
Typhoid	5–6	10–12
Phase I	14–16	15
Phase II	18–20	25
Paratyphoid B vaccine	Uninterrupted (peak outbursts lasting up to 10 sec)	30–35–40 90–100
Dysentery	10–15 (single and group outbursts)	10–15
Staphylococci	Reaction lasts 5–8 min (similar to other antigens)	
Type A	Fast or in single groups	Low
Type B	Slow oscillations	High
Control solution	(Only negligible alterations)	No change

[a] From Gordienko AN, Kiseleva VI, Saakov BA, Let'en AV: Electrophysiological phenomena in the nerve following action of antigens on the skin receptors. In Gordienko AN (ed): *Control of Immunogenesis by the Nervous System.* Washington, DC, National Technical Information Service, 1958, pp 22–27 (63).
[b] Injected intradermically after hexenal narcosis (isolation) of the nerve.

iologic solution, and except for some minute changes in oscillations, there were no visible bioelectric aberrations. In contrast, when typhoid, paratyphoid B or the dysentery vaccines, or staphylococci were injected near the lateral femoral cutaneous or auricular nerves, specific and dramatic changes in the normal bioelectric frequencies and amplitudes of the action potentials were recorded.

These findings offered dramatic and visible proof that the nervous system is capable of differentiating between various antigenic stimuli and have lent further credibility to the hypothesis that antibody formation may be mediated by the nervous system. After years of research, Gordienko (64) concluded:

1. As foreign microorganisms pass receptors, the irritation results in specific changes in bioelectric potentials from the involved afferent nerve. The body reacts to these stimuli by mobilizing leukocytes and synthesizing antibody.
2. Endless possibilities for the kind of "warning" that the nervous system may receive are effected by utilization of conduction velocities of various fiber types in combination with the rate of stimulation of fibers.
3. The action of receptors, afferent fibers, and the central nervous system is specific with regard to control of immunogenesis.

The possibility that the nervous system influences leukocyte distribution and/or mobilization also has been explored by Gordienko et al. (64) and others. In a study of splanchnoperipheral balance during chill and fever, Peterson and Müller (65) demonstrated the possibility that the nervous system influences leukocyte distribution. In their study, unanesthetized normal dogs were given continuous injections of small amounts of suspensions of living colibacilli with use of the Woodyatt pump. In this study, approximately 4 to 5 million organisms/cc were injected every minute. Lymph, muscle, and rectal temperature, constant leukocyte counts, and control of blood chemistry were observed. The authors hypothesized that the chill produced in dogs by the continuous injection of colibacilli was associated with increased splanchnic activity and temperatures. They hypothesized but could not demonstrate conclusively a mechanism whereby bacteria, entering the blood stream, are fixed by reticuloendothelial elements (the concept of a reticuloendothelial system is no longer considered valid (14)) in the splanchnic area. According to these authors, this mechanism causes stimulation of these cells and the organs nearby (i.e., the liver, spleen, stomach, etc.) via the sympathetic nervous system. They further hypothesized that sympathetic stimulation throughout the periphery gave rise to the muscle tremor, blood vessel constriction, and refocus of circulation to the splanchnic area involved, which is seen in chill and fever. As early as 1927, their findings indicated that the autonomic nervous system may play a role in maintaining splanchnoperipheral balance during the course of infectious diseases, particularly during chill and fever. Their findings were not considered conclusive, however. If radioactive tracer had been available to them, they could have demonstrated whether or not the bacteria were indeed fixed in the splanchnic area.

In a similar study, Arquin (66) studied the leukocyte counts in dogs and humans throughout active hunger contractions. From the experiments he determined that stomach tonus is directly related to specific fluctuations in the peripheral leukocyte counts. He believed that dilatation of the stomach following intramuscular injection of a nonspecific milk preparation was only part of a larger splanchnic response. Such dilatation in his experiments was accompanied by peripheral leukopenia, while gastric contraction was associated with peripheral leukocytosis. His study was thus in accord with the findings of Peterson and Müller. One immunologist I questioned concerning this and other studies suggested that the "chemistry" that causes hunger contractions also may affect the balance of peripheral leukocytes. If this were true, stomach tonus and peripheral leukocyte balance may not necessarily be linked in a cause-effect relationship. Physiologists believe, however, that "hunger contractions" result from a decrease in blood glucose circulating through the lateral hypothalamus (i.e., the so-called *hunger center*). In addition, the amygdala and cortical areas of the limbic system (including infraorbital regions, the hippocampal gyrus, and the cingulate gyrus) have been implicated with regulation of the hunger response. The only "chemistry" that could possibly mediate this balance would have to be blood glucose. It certainly appears more credible that the nervous system participates in this response by some unknown pathways (neuroendocrine?). Kuntz (59, 60) held that the nervous system is probably the regulator of leukocyte distribution.

Anterior Hypothalamus and Immunologic Competence

More recently, a number of articles have appeared that tend to support an anterior hypothalamic-immune connection and that suggest that the central nervous system is functional in antibody formation, hypersensitivity, and anaphylactic responses.

Lowered histamine sensitivity following spinal cord section was shown by Cooper (76). It was suggested by Stein et al. (44), however, that this was more likely a secondary effect of peripheral disturbances in blood circulation and temperature control. Hence, Stanton et al. (77) demonstrated that spinal cord section in rats depressed the hemolysin response but that the depression of this response was prevented by maintaining the animals at correct body temperature.

The hypothalamus has been connected with the anaphylactic reaction by a number of researchers (44, 45, 78, 83). Recently, Stein et al. (44) were able to demonstrate lowered titers of circulating antibody ($p < 0.01$), significant protection against lethal anaphylaxis ($p < 0.001$), and depressed delayed hypersensitivity reactions in animals with electrolytic lesions in the anterior basal hypothalamus. Male Hartley guinea pigs were utilized by these researchers. Bilateral electrolytic lesions were induced in the anterior, median, or posterior basal hypothalamus of various guinea pigs. Other guinea pigs were operated on but not lesioned (sham operated) or were not operated on at all (to act as controls). Each group was initially sensitized to picryl chloride (a hapten), which acted as an antigenic stimulus, 1 week after the operation. In each of the groups of guinea pigs, delayed cutaneous reactions to picryl chloride and tuberculin (purified protein derivative) were studied. In addition, agglutinin titers to picryl chloride hapten were taken to detect the level of circulating antibodies, and anaphylaxis reactions were recorded for each group.

That anaphylaxis occurred in 71% of the control animals and in only 18% of the guinea pigs with anterior hypothalamic lesions was taken as strong evidence that this brain center plays an important role in the reaction (44). Agglutinin titers for antibody to the picryl chloride were fully four times higher in the control guinea pigs than in the hypothalamically lesioned guinea pigs. Skin test reactions to picryl chloride and tuberculin were significantly diminished in animals with anterior hypothalamic lesions. These delayed hypersensitivity reactions were more intense in the nonoperated and sham-operated control groups. Median and posterior hypothalamic lesions, however, had no significant effect on lethal anaphylaxis, circulating antibody to the picryl chloride hapten, or delayed hypersensitivity reactions.

Further *in vitro* studies of the anterior hypothalamic-immune connection were undertaken recently by Schiavi et al. (78). Conclusions from these investigations suggested that the mechanism whereby anterior hypothalamic lesions reduce antibody titer may be via interference with antibody binding to host tissue, via modification of the antigen-antibody reaction, or via alteration of the content and release of histamine and other vasoactive substances. Finally, it was suggested that this lesion may alter the normal responsiveness of target tissues to the substances released by the antigen-antibody union (78). Thus, this hypothalamic-immune connection is the most likely explanation for the effects of psychosocial factors in decreasing the immune response in animals (see "Neuroendocrine-Immune Connection" in this chapter) and thereby in increasing the susceptibility of these animals to various viruses and bacteria as well as to neoplasias, leukemias, and cancers (44).

In an extensive review of the literature in 1981, Solomon and Amkraut (37) discussed the history of psychoimmunology and detailed specific studies, including Soviet work, that identified a specific portion of the dorsal hypothalamus of rabbits which when ablated led to complete suppression of the primary antibody response. Prolonged retention of antigen in the blood, inability to induce streptococcal antigen myocarditis, and prolonged graft retention also were effected by dorsal hypothalamic destruction (of specific nuclei), while an enhanced antibody response was seen with electrical stimulation of the same nuclei. They cited other Soviet work which again suggested a direct role of hypothalamic regulation of immune responsivity. Specifically, the firing rates of neurons (as determined by implanted electrodes) of specific hypothalamic nuclei significantly increased after immunization; this, of course, was suggestive of a feedback loop between the immune and nervous systems.

Brooks et al. (36) found that bilateral electrolytic lesions of specific limbic nuclei show *in vitro* alterations in lymphoid cell number and in lymphocyte activation in rats. Induced by concanavalin A, splenocytes decreased in number after anterior hypothalamic, ventromedial hypothalamic, and mamillary body lesioning. The number of thymocytes decreased after anterior hypothalamic lesioning but increased after hippocampal lesioning. Spleen cell responsiveness to concanavalin A decreased after anterior hypothalamic lesioning but was enhanced after mamillary body, hippocampal, and amygdaloid lesioning. Furthermore, thymocyte mitogen reactivity was enhanced by lesions of the hippocampus and amygdaloid complex. The authors concluded that the neuroendocrine system was most likely responsible for the effects, which were greatest 4 days after lesioning; thymocyte mitogen reactivity and spleen cell responsiveness returned to normal levels within 14 days. They suggested that neuroimmunomodulation is mediated by the interaction of specific hormones with specific surface receptors, which alters intrinsic lymphocyte function. They raised the question, however, of a functional anatomical link between the CNS and the immune system.

Certainly, there is other evidence to suggest that this is a valid conclusion. Nayar et al. (84) have shown that transection of sympathetic nerve can induce tumor-like growths in the salivary glands, reservoirs, gastric coeca, and midgut of the cockroach. Stein-Werblowsky (47) demonstrated that chemical sympathectomy increases the receptivity of tissues to grafts of tumor and/or phosphorylcholine conjugates. Injections of 0.5 ml tumor suspension intraperitoneally resulted in tumors in 24 of 38 sympathectomized (viz., 0.7 ml of 50% ethanol injected into the left paravertebral region) rats; only 1 of 30 intact rats developed tumor. Furthermore, in animals sacrificed as soon as the tumor became palpable, the growths appeared to be confined to the left side, which would normally be innervated by the left sympathetic chain. In another set of experiments it was shown that chemical sympathectomy had no effect on "take" of tumor in immune rats. From these experiments Stein-Werblowsky (47) concluded that the sympathetic nerves are concerned only with *initiation* of the immune or inflammatory reaction and that they set off a series of reactions leading to cell-mediated, homograft immunity. In his experiment the secondary immune response appeared to be independent of sympathetic influence.

Sympathetic influence on mild, nonlethal bile-induced pancreatitis has been demonstrated by Gilsdorf et al. (85). Increased sympathetic nervous system activity (viz., electrical stimulation of celiac ganglion) in the presence of nonlethal bile reflux pancreatitis (viz., 1 cc of 10% bile infused into the pancreatic duct) induced severe pancreatitis in 13 of 20 animals and mild pancreatitis in 2 more. In contrast, only 2 of the 12 animals without the sympathetic stimulation developed severe pancreatitis; the other 10 did not develop pancreatitis. Another series demonstrated that ablation of the anterior hypothalamus had a similar effect of inducing severe lethal necrotizing pancreatitis from a mild, nonlethal bile-induced form.

Exactly how sympathetic influences alter immune responses remains to be seen. Stein-Werblowsky (47) appeared to favor a two-stage mechanism in which an initiating agent such as a neurotropic substance precedes the promoting agent. He predicted that the high incidence of lung cancer among cigarette smokers may be due to such a mechanism. In cigarette smokers who develop lung cancer, the initiating agent may be the nicotine (which blocks the sympathetic ganglia) and the promoting agent may be the benzpyrene found in tobacco tar.

It is exceedingly more difficult to explain the role of the anterior hypothalamus in immunologic competence and, specifically, the humoral immune response. Numerous investigators (44, 45, 47, 48, 54, 78; 83) have shown that the lesions to this brain center provide protection against lethal anaphylaxis, cause depressed delayed hypersensitivity, and result in lower titers of circulating antibody. In view of modern immunologic research, some neuroendocrine mechanism(s) may be involved (9–19, 42, 43, 49–53, 75). Stein et al. (44) have proposed several mechanisms. The anterior hypothalamus is involved in regulation of secretion of thyroid-stimulating hormone (TSH), and it is known that this hormone is beneficial to the immune response (44, 50). Beyond a neuroendocrine mechanism, a functional anatomical link between the CNS and the immune system is a possibility, and evidence that the CNS is a regulator of thymic activity strongly supports this view (36, 37, 86–90).

The anterior hypothalamus has been purported to play an important role in immunologic competence, which may explain neural mediation of psychosocial stress in humans. By this route, environmental and social stresses can reduce a person's resistance to disease, leukemias, infections, and even cancer (37, 44). It is noteworthy that a similar pathway has been found for the effects of psychosocial stress on atherosclerosis. In this regard, Gutstein et al. (91) have demonstrated that electrical stimulation of the lateral hypothalamus resulted in atherosclerotic lesions in rats. Their findings suggested that even in the absence of coexisting hypercholesterolemia or hypertension, either by direct neural transmission affecting the vascular wall or by elaboration of arteriopathic substances (e.g., angiotensin II) in extravascular sites, a neural mechanism may be involved.

Vertebral Lesions and Immunologic Competence

Early evidence that vertebral lesions could be directly linked to immunologic competence in humans was presented by Speransky (57) who studied experimental and clinical cases of lobar pneumonia. Patients with viral pneumonia complaining of interscapular pain were treated by accepted medical procedures or by antibiotic therapy and injection of procaine into the interscapular paravertebral musculature. Patients who received the additional procaine injections were found to have significantly decreased morbidity and mortality.

Osteopathic studies on this question were raised early in this century by Deason (79) in an experimental study of filariasis. The study actually began by accident, when a number of Rhesus monkeys showed signs of the disease after being received for study at the A. T. Still Research Institute in Chicago. The infectious microfilaria were found in the blood, lymph, cerebrospinal fluid, nasal discharges, urine, and fecal discharges of the affected monkeys. Clinical signs included diarrhea, loss of weight, and stupor. The temperature in the infected animals ranged from subnormal to 104° F. The blood and urine pictures were considered diagnostic. Seven monkeys were treated by drug therapy alone, including magnesium sulfate and thymol (then considered to be an anthelmintic) (0.1 gm every 2 hours), and all failed to recover. Seven of 14 animals treated by correction of vertebral lesions by osteopathic manipulation in addition to drug therapy made complete recoveries, and another 6 showed signs of partial recovery before they died (3 of the deaths were probably due to secondary complications of pneumonia or tuberculosis).

In addition to correcting spinal lesions, osteopaths stimulate lymphatic drainage as well as venous and arterial circulation in patients with various infections (80). According to osteopathic records, during the pandemic of 1918, of 100,000 patients with influenza treated by osteopathic methods, the mortality rate was 0.25% (or 10% if deaths due to the complication of pneumonia are included), while the overall mortality rate at that time was 5% (or 30% to 60% if deaths due to the complication of pneumonia are included) (80). Modern osteopathic treatment includes the utilization of Chapman's reflexes (i.e., viscerosomatic reflexes from the liver, spleen, and adrenal cortex; certain points anterior and posterior to these organs may display overreaction or underreaction of the corresponding organ) to evaluate and/or stimulate certain viscera (80). These points are stimulated by circular friction massage for 20 to 40 seconds; according to osteopathic literature, these points correspond highly to acupuncture meridians (80).

Few studies, however, directly link vertebral lesions with immunologic competence. The works of Gordienko, Selye, Stein, Schiavi, Cooper and others, as presented in this chapter, appear to suggest that such a connection is likely. This connection should be an important area for future research, especially for chiropractors and osteopaths.

Discussion

The concept of immunity in humans is a multifaceted one, not easily understood. The variety of viewpoints involved, and the limitations on our understanding of the subject make dogmatic positions untenable. We may simplify the problem, however, by separating the various positions into two principal groups.

Traditional medical thought held that immunity was completely independent of neural influence, direct or indirect. In this model, the thymus (previously thought to be independent of neural regulation) was given an important role, and *in vitro* suppression and enhancement of classical precipitin and other immunological reactions led investigators to believe immune function was largely the result of complicated but random chemical reactions. In this model, the antigen of invading microorganisms was matched up to receptor sites on certain T cell lymphocytes that triggered an immune response (3, 5–24, 55, 92, 93).

Even the lowly earthworm, sea star, and sea urchin (*Lytechinus pictus*), which are invertebrates, have adaptive immunity (93). In fact, the sea urchin *L. pictus* has a highly sensitive immune system capable of rejecting allografts from unrelated sea urchins in only 30 days. This rejection time is even more amazing when one considers the low metabolic temperature of these animals (15 to 20° C). The experiments on *Lytechinus* support the theory of transplantation (viz., that antigenic differences of graft tissues are recognized as foreign to the host and subsequently are rejected) and demonstrate that complicated immune responses can occur in the absence of a nervous system similar to that of *homo sapiens.*

If complicated immunological responses can occur in the absence of a nervous system, however, it must also be acknowledged that complicated immune reactions can be suppressed in the presence of a nervous system. Moreover, immunosuppression clearly can be the result of direct or at least indirect neural influence. Hence, hypnotic-induced inhibition of an allergic reaction (urticarial skin test) as well as enhancement can be demonstrated despite the presence of antibodies in the sera (IgE), as documented by the allergic reaction in nonallergic volunteers who received sera from the hypnotized patients (34).

Present medical thought, however, holds that immunity is indirectly influenced by neuroendocrine factors and, possibly, by direct neural modulation. A growing number of researchers (36–38, 44–48, 54, 56–66, 78–85) now hold that the nervous system plays an important role in signaling the onset of invasion by microorganisms, by participating in some way with at least the primary immune response and, principally, by participating in the humoral immune response. Their research to some degree is supported by an overwhelming amount of evidence that now links the nervous system to immunity by way of its control of endocrine function (34–43, 49–53, 75–77, 86–89, 94). Even the thymus, once thought to be free of neural influence, has now been shown to be influenced directly by CNS activity (87).

In fact, it is probably fair to say that nearly all immunologists now recognize some role for the nervous system in modulating immune system function. Whether there is a direct neural role for initiating an immune response remains to be seen; the nervous system must have some way of modifying immunological function in the presence of psychosocial stresses, however, as there is now clearly convincing evidence for such an effect.

What is important for the chiropractic profession is that regardless of the specific mechanisms involved, there are pathways for neural modulation of immunologic competence. If psychosocial stresses can influence immunologic competence by acting through neuroendocrine or direct neural mechanisms, why couldn't the intervertebral subluxation? Reviews of medical studies throughout this book have shown that the effects of the intervertebral subluxation are wide ranging, in some cases possibly altering neural transmission, vertebral artery supply, axoplasmic transport and somatoautonomic neural traffic. The possibility that one or more of these effects may alter hypothalamic function is distinct (e.g., vertebral arteries provide a major portion of the blood supply to the brain stem and hypothalamus; see also Chapter 9). In this way endocrine and immune function might possibly be affected by intervertebral subluxations.

It is particularly gratifying that our profession's much maligned founders (D. D. Palmer has been called a "grocer and magnetic healer" by our detractors) were 80 years ahead of the time with regard to the basic emphasis they placed on neural influence of all body functions, including immunity. Of course, we now recognize other factors and the role that they too play in health and disease, but then to some degree so did the Palmers. D. D. Palmer spoke of altered tonus, and B. J. Palmer spoke of "dis-ease" or the lack of organized function or relative health (1, 67, 95). If there is any doubt that the chiropractic *neurodystrophic hypothesis*, i.e., "that neural dysfunction is stressful to the visceral and other body structures, and that this 'lowered tissue resistance' can modify the nonspecific and specific immune responses, and alter the trophic function of the involved nerves," is not a valid clinical research hypothesis, it also remains to be demonstrated as to how neuroendocrine function can alter immunologic competence. There simply can be no question that the autonomic nervous system regulates directly and indirectly the functions of all organs and tissues and influences even biochemical processes at the cellular and subcellular level (35, 40). That this trophic influence can affect "innate resistance" in humans, as the Palmers stated, is no longer purely speculative. Moreover, the issue now is more a chiropractic clinical one (i.e., proof that intervertebral subluxations in humans affect immune system function).

There is some recent research that links the vertebral lesion to alteration of immunological competence. Vora and Bates (94) at Northwestern College of Chiropractic were able to demonstrate significantly increased B cell lymphocytes following 4 weeks of twice weekly spinal manipulations in patients known to have radiographically demonstrable spinal lesions. Unfortunately, the number of patients studied was small, and more research in this area is indicated. The question remains, "To what degree might the vertebral lesion act as a neuroendocrine-immune stressor?" Whether or not this mechanism plays a significant role or merely a modest role in health remains to be determined.

Nevertheless, in the final analysis the nervous system in humans does appear to play an important and functional role in immunological competence. It seems reasonable to assume that postural and musculoskeletal abnormalities can affect this neural role in much the same way as psychic stressors (high-pitched tones) caused mice to become more susceptible to tumor-take, as well as viral and bacterial infections (44).

Summary

This chapter has focused on the role of the nervous system in immunologic competence and on the possibility of its derangement in the presence of intervertebral subluxation. It is known that primary and secondary immune responses can be demonstrated and inhibited *in vitro* (5–9). This fact and the majority of traditional immunological research have suggested that the immune response in humans is largely independent of neural influence (3, 5–24, 92, 93). The founder of chiropractic, however, believed that irritated nerves would result in "lowered tissue resistance" (1). The *neurodystrophic hypothesis*, i.e., "that neural dysfunction is stressful to the visceral and other body structures, and that this 'lowered tissue resistance' can modify the nonspecific and specific immune responses, and alter the trophic function of the involved nerves," was developed from his early writings. Psychoneuroimmunologic research of the past decade has identified a strong relationship between CNS function and immunologic competence (34–41). Some of these researchers and others

(39–41, 56–66, 75–86) have concluded that the nervous system is intimately involved in specific and nonspecific body defenses. Not only has a connection between portions of the hypothalamus and immune responses been established, but also a functional anatomical link between the thymus and the CNS has been identified (36, 37, 86–90). Other researchers have identified what they believe is a mechanism whereby the nervous system signals, guides, and directs the immune response (37, 56–64). There is overwhelming evidence to support the chiropractic *neurodystrophic hypothesis*, but there is scant evidence to directly link the vertebral lesion with immunologic competence in human clinical studies.

References

1. Palmer DD: *The Science, Art and Philosophy of Chiropractic.* Portland, OR, Portland Printing House, 1910, p 19.
2. Editors: *Chiropractic: The Unscientific Cult.* Chicago, AMA Department of Investigation, 1966.
3. Botta JR (ed): Chiropractors healers or quacks? Part 1: the 80-year war with science. *Consumer Rep* 40:542–547, 1975.
4. Botta JR (ed): Chiropractors healers or quacks? Part 2: how chiropractors can help— or harm. *Consumer Rep* 40:606–610, 1975.
5. Frobisher M, Fuerst R: *Microbiology in Health and Disease.* Philadelphia, Saunders, 1973, pp 275–309.
6. Roitt IM: *Essential Immunology.* Oxford, Blackwell, 1974, pp 1–19, 43–82, 86–94, and 166.
7. Freedman SO, Gold P: *Clinical Immunology.* Hagerstown, MD, Harper & Row, 1976.
8. Hobart MJ, McConnell I: *The Immune System.* Oxford, Blackwell, 1975.
9. Frelinger JA, Niederhuber JE, Schreffler DC: Inhibition of immune responses *in vitro* by specific antiserums to Ia antigens. *Science* 188:268–270, 1975.
10. Editors: Spotting invaders: Which cells decide? *Sci News* 111:358, 1977.
11. Burnet FM: *The Clonal Selection Theory of Acquired Immunity.* Nashville, Vanderbilt University Press, 1959, pp 49–68.
12. Volpe EP, Turpen JB: Thymus: central role in the immune system of the frog. *Science* 190:1101–1103, 1975.
13. Chandra RK: Antibody formation in first and second generation offspring of nutritionally deprived rats. *Science* 190:289–290, 1975.
14. Mogensen S: Role of macrophages in natural resistance to virus infections. *Microbiol Rev* 43:1–26, 1979.
15. Romagnani S, Maggi E, Lorenzini M, Giudizi GM, Biagiotti R, Ricci M: Study of some properties of the receptor for IgM on human lymphocytes. *Clin Exp Immunol* 36:502–510, 1979.
16. Yodoi J, et al: Lymphocytes bearing Fc receptors for IgE. *J Immunol* 123:455–460, 1979.
17. Fundenberg HH (ed): *Basic and Clinical Immunology.* Los Altos, CA, Lange, 1976.
18. Gell PGH, et al: *Clinical Aspects of Immunology.* Oxford, Blackwell, 1975.
19. Roberts NJ, Douglas RG, Simons RM, Diamond ME: Virus-induced interferon produc-

tion by human macrophages. *J Immunol* 123:365–369, 1979.
20. Patterson R: *Allergic Diseases.* Philadelphia, Lippincott, 1972.
21. Raffel S: *Immunity, Hypersensitivity, Serology.* New York, Appleton-Century-Crofts, 1953.
22. Samter M (ed): *Immunological Diseases.* Boston, Little, Brown & Co, 1971.
23. Setcarz FE (ed): *The Immune System.* New York, Academic Press, 1974.
24. Editors: Antibody construction. *Sci Dig* 16–17, December 1975.
25. Illich I: *Medical Nemesis.* New York, Bantam, 1977.
26. Grant M: *Handbook of Community Health.* Philadelphia, Lea & Febiger, 1975.
27. Honorof I, McBean E: *Vaccination the Silent Killer.* Sherman Oaks, CA, Honor Publications, 1977.
28. Wilson G: *The Hazards of Immunization.* London, Athlone Press, 1967.
29. Mendelsohn R: To immunize or not? It's a puzzler (nationally syndicated column). *Des Moines Sunday Register,* 4E, January 1, 1978.
30. Kotulak R: Dormant antiviral vaccines may be trouble years later. *Chicago Tribune,* March 31, 1975.
31. De Long R: Genetic manipulation. *Sci News* July 31, 1976.
32. Restak R: Meat cleaver or scalpel. *Saturday Rev* November 26, 1976.
33. Editors: Government using deception to sell vaccination program. *Caveat Emptor* 6:264, 1976.
34. Hall HR: Hypnosis and the immune system: a review with implications for cancer and the psychology of healing. *Am J Clin Hypn* 25:92–103, 1983.
35. Gurkalo VK, Zabezhinski MA: On participation of the autonomic nervous system in the mechanisms of chemical carcinogenesis. *Neoplasma* 29:301–307, 1982.
36. Brooks WH, Cross RJ, Roszman TL, Markesbery WR: Neuroimmunomodulation: Neural anatomical basis for impairment and facilitation. *Ann Neurol* 12:56–61, 1982.
37. Solomon GF, Amkraut AA: Psychoneuroendocrinological effects on the immune response. *Ann Rev Microbiol* 35:155–184, 1981.
38. Keller SE, Weiss JM, Schleifer SJ, Miller NE, Stein M: Suppression of immunity by stress: Effect of a graded series of stressors on lymphocyte stimulation in the rat. *Science* 213:1397–1400, 1981.
39. Locke SE: Stress, adaptation, and immunity: Studies in humans. *Gen Hosp Psychiatr* 4:49–58, 1982.
40. Guth L: "Trophic" influences of nerve on muscle. *Physiol Rev* 48:645–687, 1968.
41. Riley V: Psychoneuroendocrine influences on immunocompetence and neoplasia. *Science* 212:1100–1109, 1981.
42. Selye H, Heuser G (eds): *Fifth Annual Report on Stress.* New York, MD Publications, 1956, pp 25–63.
43. Selye H: *Stress and Disease.* New York, McGraw-Hill, 1956.
44. Stein M, Schiavi RC, Camerino M: Influence of brain and behavior on the immune system. *Science* 191:435–440, 1976.
45. Macris MT, Schiavi RC, Camerino MS, Stein M: Effect of hypothalamic lesions on immune processes in the guinea pig. *Am J Physiol* 219:1205–1209, 1970.
46. Greenspan J, Melchior J: The effect of osteopathic manipulative treatment on the resistance of rats to stressful situations. *J Am Osteopath Assoc* 65:87–91, 1966.
47. Stein-Werblowsky R: The sympathetic nervous system and cancer. *Exp Neurol* 42:97–100, 1974.
48. Editors: Social stress and the immune system. *Sci News* 107:68–69, 1975.
49. Fabris N, Pierpaoli W, Sorkin E: Lymphocytes, hormones and ageing. *Nature* 240:557–559, 1972.
50. Denckla WD: Interactions between age and the neuroendocrine and immune systems. *Fed Proc* 37:1263–1267, 1978.

51. Bilder GE, Denckla WD: Restoration of ability to reject xenografts and clear carbon after hypophysectomy of adult rats. *Mech Ageing Dev* 6:153–163, 1977.

52. Van Dijk H, Jacobse-Geels H: Evidence for the involvement of corticosterone in the ontogeny of the cellular immune apparatus of the mouse. *Immunology* 35:637–642, 1978.

53. Settipane GA, Pudupakkam RK, McGowan JH: Corticosteroid effect on immunoglobulins. *J Allergy Clin Immunol* 62:162–166, 1978.

54. Monjan AA, Collector MI: Stress-induced modulation of the immune response. *Science* 196:307–308, 1977

55. Murphy HM, Wideman CH, Brown TS: Plasma corticosterone levels and ulcer formation in rats with hippocampal lesion. *Neuroendocrinology* 28:123–130, 1979.

56. Speransky AD: *A Basis for the Theory of Medicine.* Leningrad, International Publications, 1943, pp 144–160.

57. Speransky AD: Experimental and lobar pneumonia. *Am Rev Soviet Med* 2:22–27, 1944.

58. Kuntz A: Anatomic and physiologic properties of the cutaneo-visceral vasomotor reflex arc. *J Neurophysiol* 1945.

59. Kuntz A, Haselwood LA: Circulatory reactions in the gastrointestinal tract elicited by local cutaneous stimulation. *Am Heart J* 20:743–749, 1940.

60. Kuntz A: *Autonomic Nervous System.* Philadelphia, Lea & Febiger, 1945.

61. Gordienko AN, Tsynkalovskii RB, Saakov BA, Karnitskaya NV: Reflex mechanism of antibody production following intracutaneous administration of antigen with subsequent removal of antigen depot. In Gordienko AN (ed): *Control of Immunogenesis by the Nervous System.* Washington, DC, National Technical Information Service, 1958, pp 38–43.

62. Gordienko AN, Kiseleva VI, Saakov BA, Bondarev IM, Zhigalini LI: The possibility of a reflex mechanism producing antibodies when antigen acts on skin receptors. In Gordienko AN (ed): *Control of Immunogenesis by the Nervous System.* Washington, DC, National Technical Information Service, 1958, pp 44–52.

63. Gordienko AN, Kiseleva VI, Saakov BA, Let'en AV: Electrophysiological phenomena in the nerve following action of antigens on the skin receptors. In Gordienko AN (ed): *Control of Immunogenesis by the Nervous System.* Washington, DC, National Technical Information Service, 1958, pp 22–27.

64. Gordienko AN (ed): *Control of Immunogenesis by the Nervous System.* Washington, DC, National Technical Information Service, 1958, pp 1–21.

65. Peterson WF, Müller EF: The splanchnoperipheral balance during chill and fever. *Arch Intern Med* 40:573–593, 1927.

66. Arquin S: Stomach tonus and peripheral leukocyte count (splanchnoperipheral balance). *Arch Intern Med* 41:913–923, 1928.

67. Palmer BJ: *The Subluxation Specific—The Adjustment Specific.* Davenport, IA, Palmer School of Chiropractic, 1934, pp 95–99.

68. Verner JR, Weiant CW, Watkins RJ: *Rational Bacteriology.* New York, published privately, 1953, p 204.

69. Watkins RJ: The neurology of immunization. *Ohio Chiropractic Phys Assoc,* 1–12, 1959.

70. Homewood AE: *The Neurodynamics of the Vertebral Subluxation,* ed 3. St Petersburg, FL, Valkyrie Press, 1979.

71. Carver W: *Carver's Chiropractic Analysis.* Oklahoma City, Carver Chiropractic College, 1921.

72. Watkins RJ: Principles of nerve activity. Unpublished, 1978.

73. Janse J: History of the development of chiropractic concepts; chiropractic terminology. In Goldstein M (ed): *The Research Status of Spinal Manipulative Therapy.* Washington, DC, Government Printing Office, 1975, pp 25–42.

74. Gillet H, Ward L: A discussion on spinal stress. *J Clin Chiropractic* 2:36–46, 1978.

75. Hoyrup E: Impaired adrenal function as a contributory factor in constitutional asthenia. *Acta Psychiatr Neurol [Suppl]* 107:185–196, 1956.

76. Cooper IS: A neurologic evaluation of the cutaneous histamine reaction. *J Clin Invest* 29:465–469, 1950.

77. Stanton A, Muenning L, Kopeloff LM, Kopeloff N: Spinal cord section and hemolysin-production in the rat. *J Immunol* 44:237–246, 1942.

78. Schiavi RC, Macris NT, Camerino M, Stein M: Effect of hypothalamic lesions on immediate hypersensitivity. *Am J Physiol* 228:596–601, 1975.

79. Deason J: An experimental study of filariasis. *Still Res Inst Bull* 2:191–215, 1916.

80. Rumney I: Osteopathic manipulative treatment of infectious diseases. In Stark EH (ed): *Osteopathic Medicine.* Acton, MA, Publication Sciences Group, 1975, pp 165–169.

81. Korr IM: The spinal cord as organizer of disease processes: some preliminary perspectives. *J Am Osteopath Assoc* 76:89–99, 1976.

82. Korr IM: Sustained sympathicotonia as a factor in disease. In Korr IM (ed): *The Neurobiologic Mechanisms in Manipulative Therapy.* New York, Plenum, 1978, pp 229–268.

83. Luparello TJ, Stein M, Park CD: Effect of hypothalamic lesions on rat anaphylaxis. *Am J Physiol* 207:911–914, 1964.

84. Nayar KK, Arthur E, Balls M: The transmission of tumors induced in cockroaches by nerve severance. *Experientia* 27:183–184, 1971.

85. Gilsdorf RB, Long D, Moberg A, Leonard AS: Central nervous system influence on experimentally induced pancreatitis. *JAMA* 192:134–137, 1965.

86. Kaneko M, Hiroshige T: Fast, rate-sensitive corticosteroid negative feedback during stress. *Am J Physiol* 234:R39–45, 1978.

87. Bulloch K, Moore RY: Innervation of the thymus gland by brain stem and spinal cord in mouse and rat. *Am J Anat* 162:157–166, 1981.

88. Radford HM: The effect of hypothalamic lesions on estradiol-induced changes in LH release in the ewe. *Neuroendocrinology* 28:307–312, 1979.

89. Gray GD, Smith ER, Damassa DA, Ehrenkranz JRC, Davidson JM: Neuroendocrine mechanisms mediating the suppression of circulating testosterone levels associated with chronic stress in male rats. *Neuroendocrinology* 25:247–256, 1978.

90. Follenius E, Dubois MP: Distribution of fibres reacting with an α-endorphin antiserum in the neurohypophysis of *Carassius auratus* and *Cyprinus carpio. Cell Tissue Res* 189:251–256, 1978.

91. Gutstein WH, Harrison J, Parl F, Kiu B, Avitable M: Neural factors contribute to atherogenesis. *Science* 199:449–451, 1978.

92. Bleier R, Albrecht R, Cruce JAF: Supraependymal cells of hypothalamic third ventricle: Identification as resident phagocytes of the brain. *Science* 189:299–301, 1975.

93. Coffaro KA, Hinegardner RT: Immune response in the sea urchin *Lytechinus pictus. Science* 197:1389–1390, 1977.

94. Vora GS, Bates HA: The effects of spinal manipulation on the immune system (a preliminary report). *ACA J Chiropractic* 14:S103–S105, 1980.

95. Gold RR: *The Triune of Life.* Davenport, IA, International Chiropractic Association, 1966.

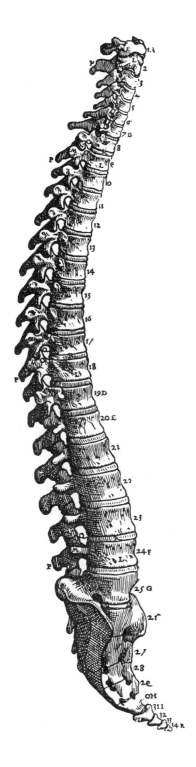

Section 3

Validating Chiropractic Theories

There is but one sure road of
access to truth—the road of
patient, cooperative inquiry
operating, by means of
observation, experiment,
record, and controlled
reflection.

John Dewey

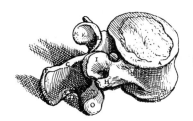

Chapter 13

Correction
of the Subluxation

*O*bjective clinical assessment of chiropractic manipulative therapy has long been the enigma of chiropractic science. Yet it is with an understanding of the logistical, economic, and medico-sociological barriers to chiropractic research that one gains a true appreciation for the great strides that chiropractic researchers have indeed made (1). Chiropractors have devised a number of specific adjustive techniques that are utilized to correct spinal and extra-spinal subluxations (2). Traditionally, chiropractic has been a method of adjusting the spine by hand only (3). Now, however, in some techniques of adjustment, instruments are utilized to deliver a thrust of controlled amplitude and duration (4, 5). The use of specific x-ray analyses is complementary to the use of precise, controlled chiropractic manipulative technique (6, 7). It should be noted that chiropractic methods of analysis are sometimes contradictory. It is hoped that computer-aided x-ray analysis of the spine, which is under study at the University of Colorado, may help to clear up some of the present confusion and contradictions (8, 9). Three-dimensional x-ray views of the spine may be part of chiropractic practice in the future (10). Evaluation of subluxation correction by use of electromyography, dynamic thermography, Moire contourography, the posturometer, and reliability studies of clinical findings has been the focus of contemporary chiropractic research efforts (11–15). These and other research efforts point to the need for controlled, blinded clinical trials to determine whether chiropractic manipulation is effective in correcting definable predetermined spinal subluxations.

Chiropractic Treatment of Musculoskeletal Disorders

Studies indicating that chiropractic care is effective in treating such disparate clinical entities as low back pain and migraine headache have been on record for some time (16–18). The controversy surrounding even medical research of chiropractic manipulation, however, is intense within both medical and chiropractic communities. Hence, the finding that 17 patients continued to be free of headache more than 1 year following chiropractic treatment prompted one medical researcher to write that the original medical diagnosis of migraine must have been wrong, since migraine headaches involved vascular and humoral changes in the cranial circulation remote from the cervical spine (19). Obviously, this researcher who ignored the role of the vertebral artery (see Chapter 9) rejected even medical research regarding the efficacy of chiropractic treatment. In a prospective and retrospective study, Vernon (20) found evidence of significant decrease in frequency, duration, and severity of headaches in patients treated by chiropractic manipulation.

Evidence that chiropractic manipulation can correct static subluxations of the spine has been provided by Grostic and DeBoer (21), Leach (22), and others utilizing retrospective inspection of radiographic films (23, 24). This evidence contrasts with research by Roberts et al. (25) who in a prospective trial of physiotherapeutic manipulation found no change in bone position by radiographic assessment.

Use of heel lifts is widespread throughout the chiropractic profession, and chiropractic investigations have been made into assessment of leg length inequality and its affect on the spine, treatment by use of heel lifts, and assessment of improvement by radiographic, electromyographic, and other means (11, 26, 27).

Fonti and Lynch (28) found that chiropractic treatment was extremely effective (84.8% excellent or good results) in 3136 cases of lumbosciatalgia caused by disc disease, in which there was protrusion but without frank herniation. All patients had previously failed pharmacotherapeutic and/or physiotherapeutic treatments. In a 2-year follow-up after 30 chiropractic treatments followed by mechanical traction, 50.4% of patients had excellent results with no painful relapses. Another 34.4% required further treatment after relapses which then responded favorably. Only 15.2% showed no significant improvement, according to this study in Italy conducted jointly by a medical doctor (orthopedist) and a doctor of chiropractic.

Crispini and Mantero (29) found that improvement in postpartal spinal pain after chiropractic was evident in 90 of 120 patients. In their study, most of the 10% who failed to respond to chiropractic had gynecologic complications (uterine inflammations, fibromas, cysts, etc.) causing reflex lumbosacral pain.

Cox (30) has studied the use of flexion distraction therapy in the treatment of intervertebral disc lesions and facet syndrome. He has demonstrated excellent recovery in 82% of 67 patients with lumbar disc protrusions and spinal stenosis.

Although there are numerous other chiropractic research studies regarding the efficacy of chiropractic treatment for various musculoskeletal disorders, few offer blinded or controlled data for inspection.

Chiropractic Treatment of Organic Disorders

There are some interesting chiropractic investigations regarding chiropractic manipulative therapy (CMT) and several organic and neurological disorders. Nearly all of the significant research in this area has been conducted since 1975. The role of CMT in the treatment of hypertension has been addressed in initial investigations by Dulgar et al. (31), Tran and Kirby (32, 33), and others (Vitelli and Leach, unpublished observations) who were able to demonstrate a hypotensive effect for chiropractic adjustment.

Initial investigations regarding CMT and its effect on the electrogastrogram suggest a relationship between gastric tone and vagal activity and upper cervical adjustment (34).

Vora and Bates (35) were able to demonstrate immune system alterations following CMT (i.e., significantly increased B lymphocytes—see Chapter 12).

Wickes (36) found evidence of significantly elevated blood pressure (systolic) in the ankle following thoracolumbar CMT.

It should be noted that all of the above-mentioned studies involved matching manipulated groups with nonmanipulated or sham-manipulated control groups (31–37). For example, in the study by Wiles (34), 13 healthy volunteers were divided into two groups; one group received chiropractic upper cervical manipulation, while the other group was only motion palpated. Significantly increased basic gastric tone ($p < 0.01$) as well as "normalization" of the wave patterns was demonstrated in manipulated patients only.

Research findings presented at the World Chiropractic Conference held in Italy in 1982 indicated that chiropractic may be of benefit in a wide variety of musculoskeletal and otovestibular symptomatology, as well as cardiovascular disorders. Reduction of lumbar, sciatic, and cervicobrachial pain was evidenced by reduced peak latencies of somatosensory evoked potentials (37). Improvement in sensory and motor function was cited in one study, and reduction of vertigo, headache, tinnitus, and visual disorders in patients with vertebrobasilar arterial insufficiency without arterial hypoplasia was reported in another (37). EMG (H reflex) studies of patients receiving chiropractic treatment for lumbosciatalgia indicated objective evidence of improvement after 30 chiropractic treatments (37). Evidence for improvement of patients with Barré's syndrome and cervical arthrosis after only 10 chiropractic adjustments was established clinically by reduced plasma levels of calcitonin, dosed by antiserum A, as well as symptomatically by reduced paresthesia, cervicalgia, headache, vertigo, and tinnitus (37).

Tonal audiometry, impedancemetry, automatic audiometry, electronystagmographic recordings, eye tracking tests, and visual suppression tests were conducted before and after chiropractic treatment in 80 patients presenting with otovestibular symptomatology (37). Chiropractic adjustments with mechanical traction resulted in improvement in otovestibular balance in virtually every patient presenting with arthrosis and static-dynamic cervical changes and symptoms including vertigo, tinnitus, and hypoacusis. In the study, conducted jointly by a medical doctor and a doctor of chiropractic, vascular disorders were investigated initially with cerebral rheography. Only in the case of hypoacusis did the majority of the patients fail to have a good to excellent response (only 19 of 59 patients with hypoacusis improved after chiropractic). In every other category, objective clinical tests demonstrated significant improvement in the majority of patients after chiropractic manipulation.

These studies collectively offer clinical evidence of somatovisceral responses and the first chiropractic clinical evidence that specific chiropractic manipulation can affect autonomic function.

Certainly, there is a great need for larger scale research efforts in this area.

One other study that should be noted was conducted in 1973 for the chiropractic profession by the Psychoeducational and Guidance Services at College Station, Texas (38). Independent investigators evaluated children with learning and behavioral impairments due to brain damage and/or neurological dysfunction and with emotional impairments. These children were referred to chiropractors for treatment. Follow-up evaluation by the diagnosticians showed that 12 of the 13 children (who had previously failed to respond to medical care) in this pilot study demonstrated some degree of improvement. The investigators concluded that chiropractic treatment "appears to be highly effective in the treatment of children with learning impairments and emotional problems." A follow-up study by these investigators (a clinical psychologist, superintendent of schools, and the director of Psychoeducational and Guidance Services) showed that the 12 students receiving chiropractic manipulation achieved reduction of hyperactivity and improved attention span and that these gains were more sustained than those in a similar group of 12 children receiving medication. The study, however, apparently lacked controls and objective evidence of change in autonomic nervous system function (such as arousal) which would have lent more credibility to the findings. Center and Leach (39) have indicated that the addition of galvanic skin response testing would have provided a measure of autonomic function and arousal and that the use of a single subject research design as a control procedure, would have been an improvement over their study design.

Another area of interest to holistic practitioners of chiropractic care is in the nutritional treatment of diseases and prevention of disease by the nutritional approach. Even Palmer (40) acknowledged that altered chemistry could cause spinal subluxations, and proponents of that hypothesis have held that treating the body nutritionally is important in keeping the body free of spinal subluxations once they have been corrected chiropractically. Hence, a significant number of chiropractic research efforts have addressed the nutrition question.

It is now an established fact that nutrition does indeed play an important role in host resistance to malignancy and resistance to disease (41–43). What is poorly understood, however, is whether muscle testing (a procedure that is commonly employed by some chiropractors and that involves testing for weakness of specific muscles by manually resisting their pull) can be used as an indicator of nutritional status. Triano (44) found no evidence that "weak" muscles or reactive muscles can be strengthened by sublingual or topical application of glandular substances. In a blinded study, substances that were alleged to increase strength of reactive muscles were found not to have any affect significantly greater than that from control substances. In a blinded trial of muscle strength testing, Rybeck and Swenson (45) were able to demonstrate significantly weakened latissimus dorsi muscle with manual testing but not with a mechanical testing device, after subjects had been administered refined sugar orally. Because of the results of these studies, the widespread use of muscle strength testing as an indicator of nutritional status, at least as these tests are currently being employed in chiropractic today, is being questioned.

There are numerous other studies in the chiropractic literature concerning the use of specific nutritional substances. For example, Miller et al. (46) found no significant change in maximal oxygen uptake in young women after heme-iron supplementation. Brown et al. (47) were unable to detect improved muscle strength or endurance after natural or synthetic vitamin E supplementation. Hogan and Kaplan (48) demonstrated a normalizing effect of magnesium orotate in lowering cholesterol and triglycerides. Davis et al. (49) were able to demonstrate that vitamin B_{12} was absorbed more effectively in a resin-bound form than in a free form. These studies are examples of nutritional research that is necessary if chiropractic is to claim a role in nutritional and holistic approach to health care. Obviously, the nutritional question is beyond the scope of this text, but the reader is urged to follow the *Journal of Manipulative and Physiological Therapeutics* and other refereed journals for objective research in this area.

Efficacy of Chiropractic Adjustment versus Medical Therapy

Studies regarding the efficacy of chiropractic care in the treatment of neck and low back strain and sprain have been undertaken (50–56). Most of these studies have compared chiropractic care with medical care.

In a study of 744 patients with neck and back pain, 70.5% were either much improved or fully recovered under chiropractic care (50). These chronic low back pain patients were largely referrals from a university hospital and general practitioners; even patients with postsurgical low back pain showed improvement.

Cox (30) achieved excellent results in 82% of 67 patients with lumbar disc lesions (40% had received prior medical care) with use of chiropractic flexion-traction and range-of-motion techniques.

Workman's compensation records from several states, which were analyzed by independent experts, reveal a remarkable trend (51–54). These records indicate that patients with back strains and sprains recover quicker and at less expense (51–54) and are more satisfied with chiropractic care than with medical care (56).

Efficacy of Medical Manipulative Procedures versus Sham and Control Therapies

Fisk (57) utilized medical manipulative procedures to obtain complete recovery in 90% of patients suffering from the acute low back pain syndrome. Fisk concluded that in these acute cases, manipulation works best only in the early course of the syndrome. Unfortunately, Fisk used no controls in his study.

In another interesting study, Glover et al. (58) utilized rotational manipulation of the trunk to correct a syndrome that they defined as including back pain, skin hyperesthesia, tenderness, and limitation of the trunk in one or more directions of movement. Control patients received detuned diathermy treatments, while experimental patients received undefined rotational manipulation (i.e., the authors did not describe how much force was utilized, what anatomical points were contacted by the manipulator, whether the patient was seated or side-lying, etc.). Statistically significant improvement was seen after the first and only manipulation. Although there was no statistical difference between the pain in both groups 7 days later, it was pointed out that follow-up manipulative procedures may have continued to produce improvement. That these were acute care cases is evidenced by the fact that all patients under 26 years of age improved completely by the end of the first week, regardless of whether or not they received manipulation.

In a multicenter study, Doran and Newell (59) compared manipulation to physiotherapy, corset application, and analgesic therapy. After 3 weeks of the therapies, 64% of those in the manipulated group, 52% of those in the physiotherapy group (who received more treatments than those in the manipulated group), and 49% and 48% of those in the corset and analgesic (Panadol) groups, respectively, reported that they were better. By inclusion of patients with slight to complete recovery, the authors noted that 75% in each group were better 3 weeks posttherapy. The authors then concluded that manipulation produces statistically significant improvement only initially (immediately after treatment). Closer analysis of the data, however, suggests that a long-term manipulative effect was demonstrated. Hence, looking at the moderately to completely relieved groups 3 weeks after treatment (with data from the "slightly better" group left out) again showed that degree of improvement was best with those who received manipulation (65%) than with those in the physiotherapy (54%) and corset/analgesic (47%) groups, respectively.

Berqquist-Ullman and Larsson (60) studied 217 industrial workers with low back pain. Only acute care patients who had no prior history of back pain within the past year were included in the study. The authors found no difference between patients treated with "back school," physiotherapy, or placebo short-wave diathermy at the lowest possible setting. The results from manipulation were not utilized.

Haldeman (61) found that spinal exercise benefits patients with low back pain. He could not demonstrate, however, a complete recovery with this regimen in most patients.

Sloop et al. (62) were unable to demonstrate a beneficial effect for a single manipulation of the neck in anesthetized patients with chronic neck pain. The authors did admit, however, that while they could not find a "consistent favorable response for manipulation," their tests did favor patients in the manipulated group.

According to medical doctors in Great Britain who practice manipulation, this treatment has been used to successfully correct mild vertebrobasilar artery ischemic attacks causing giddiness or dizziness (63). These doctors also used atlantal manipulation to successfully correct another vertebrobasilar disorder of the neck (see also Chapter 9).

Sims-Williams et al. (64) were not able to demonstrate improvement in chronic low back pain patients after 4 weeks of Maitlandtype mobilization and manipulation, compared with a control group receiving detuned diathermy placebo treatments. They concluded that manipulation would not help patients with chronic and severe low back pain.

Jayson et al. (65) discussed the long-term follow-up analysis of two large studies on manipulation. They found a slight but definite improvement in the manipulated group only immediately after manipulation.

Hoehler and Tobis (66) found that the only significant test for evaluation of the effectiveness of spinal manipulative therapy (i.e., significant for interobserver reliability, low back pain, and improvement after successful spinal manipulation) was the straight leg raising (voluntary) test. Other researchers (67–69) have pointed out the importance of reliable diagnosis of low back pain patients.

Discussion

Chiropractic clinical research has shown promise in validating chiropractic hypotheses by demonstrating clinical improvement in some patients with musculoskeletal and organic disorders and diseases. This improvement suggests, therefore, that correction of the subluxation is possible clinically. Unfortunately for chiropractic researchers, the work has just begun.

Initial and pilot studies of chiropractic care for the treatment of migraine, static subluxations, hypolordosis of the cervical spine, intervertebral disc syndrome, back sprain and strain, hypertension, and hyperactivity have been carried out. Joint medical and chiropractic research on a variety of organic disorders from otovestibular symptomatology to cardiovascular disorders has yielded impressive results. These and other studies indicating a chiropractic manipulative effect on differing parameters of autonomic function provide only a background for more extensive research that will verify these findings, target specific conditions and types of subluxation that respond best to manipulation, and provide the clinician with diagnostic and prognostic information critical to the practice of chiropractic. Similarly, studies of specific nutrients and glandulars and their effects and of the role of muscle testing for nutrient analysis must be verified or cast out of clinical practice.

Although, in general, medical studies discount the efficacy of physiotherapeutic manipulation, these trials make several inaccurate assumptions; i.e., that all manipulators are alike and produce similar results; that all manipulative techniques are alike and produce similar results; and that there are single theories and techniques involved in chiropractic, physiotherapy, and osteopathy. Obviously, conclusions drawn from research with such critical design flaws may, at best, be inapplicable to chiropractic (70).

Although some researchers want research carried out on the cause or causes of back pain before research is carried out on spinal manipulation, others acknowledge that comparative research is necessary now, since 70% to 80% of the population has been shown to suffer from low back pain (71, 72). The conditions that may be responsible for low back pain include but are not limited to osteoporosis, spondylosis (Figure 13.1), subluxation, disc herniation, referred pain from visceral sources, sacralization

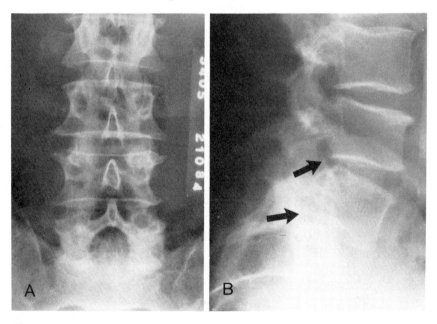

Figure 13.1. Intervertebral subluxation of L4–L5 and L5–S1 segments (*arrows*) with osteophytes and signs of degenerative joint disease. Such alterations are suggestive of a developing *spondylosis* and predispose to episodes of low back pain. Note that the AP view (*A*) demonstrates osteophytic projections at the L3 and the L4 level. In the lateral view of the lumbar spine (*B*), sclerosis of the vertebral end plates is especially noticeable at the anterior superior margin of L4. Such changes are often the result of trauma, chronic unreduced subluxation with mechanical imbalance, etc.

and lumbarization, "unstable vertebrae," fixation, congenital asymmetry, and rheumatoid arthritis or osteoarthritis (see also Appendix). Obviously, because so many causative factors must be considered in the pathogenesis of low back pain, research is made extremely complicated.

Haldeman (73) has made an extensive review of the literature with regard to specific conditions that medical manipulators have found that respond to manipulation. These musculoskeletal conditions have not been covered in this text but should prove informative to the interested reader.

In the final analysis, it appears that the chiropractic profession must continue to produce blinded and controlled research on correction of the subluxation and the subsequent clinical response but must do so on a larger scale, if the specific goals of chiropractic research are to be met. Medical trials of manipulation simply do not meet the needs of chiropractic practitioners in terms of method design and outcome. For example, anyone in chiropractic practice knows that a patient with a 6-year history of neck pain is simply not going to be expected to improve with one adjustment (62). Similarly, chiropractic procedures involving the treatment of chronic low back pain may involve specific chiropractic manipulation, physiotherapy, an exercise regimen, and posture training. In such cases, the effects of manipulation may be enhanced by the use of these other devices substantially or disproportionately, such that testing manipulation alone may give an inadequate outcome (64). These are issues that this author believes will best be addressed by chiropractic researchers.

Summary

Chiropractors have devised a number of specific adjustive (manipulative) techniques (2). Specific analytical and clinical tools for evaluation of subluxation correction have been studied (6–15). Studies of the effect of chiropractic manipulative treatment on musculoskeletal (16–30) and organic (31–38) disorders and diseases have been carried out. The role of nutrition and muscle testing has been studied (44, 45) and is discussed in light of this research. Medical research of manipulative therapy as practiced by physiotherapists has been carried out (57–65) and is discussed along with its limited applicability to chiropractic research questions. Finally, the conclusion is reached that medical research simply cannot be expected to fulfill the needs of chiropractic practitioners and their patients. Such needs and chiropractic research goals must be met by chiropractic researchers using further, controlled blinded trials of the effects of chiropractic manipulative therapy.

References

1. Wardwell WI: The present and future role of the chiropractor. In Haldeman S (ed): *Modern Developments in the Principles and Practice of Chiropractic.* New York, Appleton-Century-Crofts, 1980, pp 25–41.
2. Kfoury PW: *Catalogue of Chiropractic Techniques.* St Louis, Logan College of Chiropractic, 1977.
3. Palmer BJ: *The Subluxation Specific—The Adjustment Specific.* Davenport, IA, Palmer School of Chiropractic, 1934.
4. Pettibon BR: *Pettibon Method of Cervical X-ray Analysis and Instrument Adjusting.* Tacoma, WA, published privately, 1968.
5. Jones DE: *The Life Cervical Adjusting Technic.* Marietta, GA, Life Chiropractic College, 1977.
6. McRae J: *Roengenometrics in Chiropractic.* Toronto, published privately, 1974.
7. Watkins RJ: Upper cervical mechanics. *Today's Chiropractic* 5:14–17, 1976.
8. Suh CH: Computer-aided spinal biomechanics. In Haldeman S (ed): *Modern Developments in the Principles and Practice of Chiropractic.* New York, Appleton-Century-Crofts, 1980, pp 143–170.
9. Suh CH: Biomechanical aspects of subluxation. In Goldstein M (ed): *The Research Status of Spinal Manipulative Therapy.* Washington, DC, Government Printing Office, 1975, pp 103–119.
10. Grostic J: Some observations on computer-aided x-ray analysis. *Int Rev Chiropractic* 33:38–41, 1979.
11. Triano JJ: Objective electromyographic evidence for use and effects of lift therapy. *J Manip Physiolog Ther* 6:13–16, 1983.
12. Spector B, Fukuda F, Kanner L, Thorschmidt E: Dynamic thermography: a reliability study. *J Manip Physiolog Ther* 4:5–10, 1981.
13. Schram SB, Hosek RS, Owens ES: Computerized paraspinal skin surface temperature scanning: a technical report. *J Manip Physiolog Ther* 5:117–121, 1982.
14. Vernon H: An assessment of the intra- and inter-reliability of the posturometer. *J Manip Physiolog Ther* 6:57–60, 1983.
15. Brand NE, Gizoni CM: Moire contourography and infrared thermography: changes resulting from chiropractic adjustments. *J Manip Physiolog Ther* 5:113–116, 1982.
16. Parker GB, Tupling H, Pryor DS: Proceedings of the Australian association of manipulative medicine. *Aust NZ J Med* 8:589, 1978.
17. Gitelman R: A chiropractic approach to biomechanical disorders of the lumbar spine and pelvis. In Haldeman S (ed): *Modern Developments in the Principles and Practice of Chiropractic.* New York, Appleton-Century-Crofts, 1980, pp 297–330.
18. Schafer RC: Neck and cervical spine injuries. In Schafer RC (ed): *Chiropractic Management of Sports and Recreational Injuries.* Baltimore, Williams & Wilkins, 1982, pp 327–350.
19. Bogduk N: Headaches and cervical manipulation. *Med J Aust* 3:65–66, 1979.
20. Vernon H: Chiropractic manipulative therapy in the treatment of headaches: a retrospective and prospective study. *J Manip Physiolog Ther* 5:109–112, 1982.

21. Grostic JD, DeBoer KF: Roentgenographic measurement of atlas laterality and rotation: a retrospective pre- and post-manipulation study. *J Manip Physiolog Ther* 5:63–71, 1982.

22. Leach RA: An evaluation of the effect of chiropractic manipulative therapy on hypolordosis of the cervical spine. *J Manip Physiolog Ther* 6:17–24, 1983.

23. Palmer BJ: *History in the Making.* Davenport, IA, Palmer School Press, 1957.

24. Gimmler J: The substantiation of chiropractic by scientific research. *J Nat Chiropractic Assoc* 20–22, July 1952.

25. Roberts GM, Roberts EE, Lloyd KN, Burke MS, Evans DP: Lumbar spinal manipulation on trial. Part 2—radiological assessment. *Rheumatol Rehabil* 17:54, 1978.

26. Giles LGF, Taylor JR: Low-back pain associated with leg length inequality. *Spine* 6:510–521, 1981.

27. DeBoer KF, Harmon RO, Savoie S, Tuttle CD: Inter- and intra-examiner reliability of leg-length differential measurement: a preliminary study. *J Manip Physiolog Ther* 6:61–66, 1983.

28. Fonti S, Lynch M: Etiopathogenesis of lumbosciatalgia due to disc disease; chiropractic treatment (statistics on 3,136 patients). In Mazzarelli J (ed): *Chiropractic: Interprofessional Research.* Torino, Italy, Edizioni Minerva Medica, 1983, pp 53–57

29. Crispini L, Mantero E: Static alterations of the pelvic, sacral, lumbar area due to pregnancy; chiropractic treatment. In Mazzarelli J (ed): *Chiropractic: Interprofessional Research.* Torino, Italy, Edizioni Minerva Medica, 1983, pp 59–68.

30. Cox JM: Low back pain: recent statistics and data on its mechanism, diagnosis and treatment from chiropractic manipulation. *ACA J Chiropractic* 13:5125–5141, 1979.

31. Dulgar G, Hill D, Sirucek A, Davis B: Evidence for a possible anti-hypertensive effect of basic technique apex contact adjusting. *ACA J Chiropractic* 14:S97–S102, 1980.

32. Tran TA, Kirby JD: The effects of upper thoracic adjustment upon the normal physiology of the heart. *ACA J Chiropractic* 11:25–28, 1977.

33. Tran TA, Kirby JD: The effects of upper cervical adjustment upon the normal physiology of the heart. *ACA J Chiropractic* 11:58–62, 1977.

34. Wiles MR: Observations on the effects of upper cervical manipulations on the electrogastrogram: a preliminary report. *J Manip Physiolog Ther* 3:226–229, 1980.

35. Vora GS, Bates HA: The effects of spinal manipulations on the immune system. *ACA J Chiropractic* 14:S103–S105, 1980.

36. Wickes D: Effects of thoracolumbar spinal manipulations on arterial flow in the lower extremity. *J Manip Physiolog Ther* 3:3–6, 1980.

37. Strang VV: *Essential Principles of Chiropractic.* Davenport, IA, Palmer College of Chiropractic, 1984, pp 65–73.

38. Walton EV: The effects of chiropractic treatment on students with learning and behavioral impairments due to neurological dysfunction. *Int Rev Chiropractic* 29:4, 5, 24–26, 1975.

39. Center DB, Leach RA: The multiple baseline across subjects design: proposed use in research. *J Manip Physiolog Ther* 7:231–236, 1984.

40. Palmer DD: *The Science, Art and Philosophy of Chiropractic.* Portland, OR, Portland Printing House, 1910.

41. Mann GV: Food intake and resistance to disease. *Lancet* 1(8180):1238–1239, 1980.

42. Chandra RK: Immune response in overnutrition. *Cancer Res* 41:3795–3796, 1981.

43. Murray J, Murray A: Toward a nutritional concept of host resistance to malignancy and intracellular infection. *Perspect Biol Med* 25:290–301, 1981.

44. Triano JJ: Muscle strength testing as a diagnostic screen for supplemental nutrition therapy: a blind study. *J Manip Physiolog Ther* 5:179–182, 1982.

45. Rybeck CH, Swenson R: The effect of oral administration of refined sugar on muscle strength. *J Manip Physiolog Ther* 3:155–61, 1980.

46. Miller E, Brown B, Gorman D: The effects of hemoglobin supplements on maximal oxygen uptake in females. *J Manip Physiolog Ther* 6:189–195, 1983.

47. Brown BS, Jolley W, Andre J: Vitamin E supplementation and changes in strength and other fitness parameters. *J Manip Physiolog Ther* 3:7–12, 1980.

48. Hogan WJ, Kaplan R: The therapeutic effect of magnesium orotate in serum lipid reduction. *J Manip Physiolog Ther* 1:27–30, 1978.

49. Davis BP, Gerstein LM, Rozeboom DL, Cranwell RW: Enhanced absorption of oral vitamin B_{12} from a resin absorbate administered to normal subjects. *J Manip Physiolog Ther* 5:123–7, 1982.

50. Potter GE: A study of 744 cases of neck and back pain treated with spinal manipulation. *J Can Chiropractic Assoc* 22:154–156, 1977.

51. Wolf CR: *Industrial Back Injury.* San Francisco, California Department of Industrial Relations, Division of Labor Statistics & Research, 1970.

52. Martin RA: *A Study of Time Loss Back Claims.* Portland, OR, Oregon Workman's Compensation Board, 1971.

53. First Research Corporation: *1956 Florida Industrial Commission Cases.* Orlando, Florida Chiropractic Association, 1960.

54. Independent studies of industrial back injuries. Submitted to *International Chiropractic Association, Washington, DC.*

55. Haldeman S: Spinal manipulative therapy. *Clin Orthop* 179:62–70, 1983.

56. Kane RL, Fischer FD, Leymaster C: Manipulating the patient: a comparison of the effectiveness of physician and chiropractic care. *Lancet* 1:1333–1336, 1974.

57. Fisk JW: An evaluation of manipulation in the treatment of the acute low back pain syndrome in general practice. In Buerger A, Tobis J (eds): *Approaches to the Validation of Manipulation Therapy.* Springfield, IL, Charles C Thomas, 1977, pp 236–270.

58. Glover JR, Morris JG, Khosla T: Back pain; a randomized clinical trial of rotational manipulation of the trunk. *Br J Ind Med* 31:59–64, 1974.

59. Doran DML, Newell DJ: Manipulation in the treatment of low back pain: a multicenter study. *Br Med J* 2:161–164, 1975.

60. Berqquist-Ullman M, Larsson U: Acute low back pain in industry. *Acta Orthop Scand [Suppl]* 170:1–117, 1977.

61. Haldeman S: Low back pain: a study of 50 patients on a group exercise program. *Physiol Can* 27:71–77, 1975.

62. Sloop PR, Smith DS, Goldenberg E, Dore D: Manipulation for chronic neck pain (a double blind study). *Spine* 7:532–535, 1982.

63. Burns R: The cervical spine in manipulative medicine. *Practitioner* 222:803–806, 1979.

64. Sims-Williams H, Jayson MIV, Young SMS, Baddeley H, Collins E: Controlled trial of mobilisation and manipulation for low back pain: hospital patients. *Br Med J* 2:1318–1320, 1979.

65. Jayson MIV, Sims-Williams H, Young S, Baddeley H, Collins E: Mobilization and manipulation for low-back pain. *Spine* 6:409–416, 1981.

66. Hoehler FK, Tobis JS: Low back pain and its treatment by spinal manipulation: measures of flexibility and asymmetry. *Rheumatol Rehabil* 21:21–26, 1982.

67. Kirkaldy-Willis WH, Hill RJ: A more precise diagnosis for low-back pain. *Spine* 4:102–109, 1979.

68. McCall IW, Park WM, O'Brien JP: Induced pain referral from posterior lumbar elements in normal subjects. *Spine* 4:441–446, 1979.

69. Ghia JN, Duncan G, Toomey TC, Mao W, Gregg JM: The pharmacologic approach in differential diagnosis of chronic pain. *Spine* 4:447–451, 1979.

70. Haldeman S: What is meant by manipulation? In Buerger A, Tobis J (eds): *Approaches to the Validation of Manipulation Therapy.* Springfield, IL, Charles C Thomas, 1977, pp 299–302.

71. Nachemson AL: The problem of low back pain. In Buerger A, Tobis J (eds): *Approaches to the Validation of Manipulation Therapy.* Springfield, IL, Charles C Thomas, 1977, pp 320–322.
72. Haldeman S: Why one cause of back pain? In Buerger A, Tobis J (eds): *Approaches to the Validation of Manipulation Therapy.* Springfield, IL, Charles C Thomas, 1977, pp 187–197.
73. Haldeman S: Spinal manipulative therapy in the management of low back pain. In Finneson BE (ed): *Low Back Pain,* ed 2. Philadelphia, Lippincott, 1980.

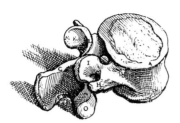

Chapter 14

Researching Chiropractic

*F*ew searches in the history of mankind have been conducted without controversy, setbacks, and frustrations. Late in the 1960s, following a personal investigation, Suh (1) concluded that the chiropractic profession needed not only broad clinical studies but also basic research. This University of Colorado professor soon came under pressure from colleagues, government officials, and health professionals to abandon the idea of initiating basic chiropractic research, even before he had begun. Yet Suh went on to organize and develop a program of study in chiropractic in areas of biomechanics, neurophysiology, and neurochemistry (2–9). These studies have been funded by the university itself, the International Chiropractors Association (ICA), the American Chiropractic Association (ACA), and the federal government.

In addition, interdisciplinary conferences in the 1970s resulted in a virtual renaissance of research for the chiropractic profession (10–13). Haldeman (14) formed "The International Society for the Advancement of Clinical Chiropractic and Spinal Research." Two other organizations, an ACA-sponsored organization, "The Foundation for Chiropractic Education and Research" (FCER), and an ICA-sponsored organization, "The Foundation for the Advancement of Chiropractic Tenets and Science" (FACTS), are based in Washington, D.C. (15, 16). An interdisciplinary chiropractic research journal, *Journal of Manipulative and Physiological Therapeutics*, has been indexed by *Index Medicus* as well as by several other scientific indexing services (17). It is also the only primary chiropractic research journal that is refereed.

The *Journal of Manipulative and Physiological Therapeutics* has provided a platform for some important chiropractic clinical research from various chiropractic college research departments and from the field. Many of these research projects have involved the use of blinds as well as controls, which overcomes flaws found

in prior chiropractic research efforts (see Chapter 13). Central to this scientific research is the concept that chiropractic can alter the natural or "normal" course of a given disease, "dis-ease", or dysfunction by correction of the intervertebral subluxation (18). For this concept to be demonstrated, the design of chiropractic studies must be objective, i.e., incorporate such fundamental procedures as multiple, double, or single blinds and employ statistically sound analyses (19). A concept that is new to chiropractic research but that is familiar to researchers in psychology and physical therapy is the use of the single subject research design, which eliminates the need for more complicated research settings (20). Utilization of such methods assures elimination of the psychosomatic factor in research which then becomes acceptable not only to other health professionals but also to the media and the public.

Approaches to Researching Chiropractic

Several major topics need intensive investigation if chiropractic tenets are to be substantiated. McDowell (18) believes that chiropractic research in the future should be directed to three primary areas: evaluation of chiropractic therapy, diagnostic technique, and relative basic science. This approach requires further division into laboratory, field, and clinical studies.

Laboratory investigations could be used to follow up on the work of Sharpless (6) and Luttges et al. (3). Such investigations are needed to determine the correlation between spinal nerve or root compression or irritation and protein and degenerative changes both proximal (spinal cord proper) and distal to the compression (see Chapter 10). Various field studies involving animals could be initiated to follow up on the work of Triano and Luttges (9). These studies are needed to determine the relationship between chronic, moderate nerve root compression or irritation (mimicking the supposed effects of subluxation) and subsequent physiological, functional, or pathological changes, if any, in the viscera. Certainly, a theoretical basis for manipulative effects on humoral immunity would be enhanced by demonstrating that ligation of upper cervical nerve roots could influence the pituitary, thyroid, or hypothalamic function known to be involved in immunity (see Chapter 12). The work of Vora and Bates (21) certainly suggests some connection between the neuroendocrine system and manipulation.

Studies of somatoautonomic phenomena as well as evidence supporting a *fixation* hypothesis (see Chapter 8) definitely need to be investigated further. It has been suggested that this theory may be the most logical justification for the use of chiropractic adjustment in the correction of conditions other than pain syndromes (22). Electromyography should prove to be an objective indicator of muscle activity in such studies, which could be performed in the solo-practitioner clinical setting. Electromyographic determination of the effects of chiropractic adjustment on muscle spasm in the dermatomes related segmentally to the viscera or function (e.g., renal secretions) to be tested could be correlated with laboratory findings to verify the relationship between the somatic and the visceral functions involved. Of course, more complicated trials could be attempted also, but it is critical that the profession determine what systemic effects, if any, result from such pheonomena as spinal fixation.

Another area deserving in-depth research involves the role of subluxation in alteration of vertebral artery blood supply to the brain stem (see Chapter 9). Some investigators have determined that this phenomenon represents a contraindication for adjustment (23, 24). The role of correction of vertebrobasilar arterial insufficiency by manipulation, if there is such a role, and the role of chiropractic adjustment in causing stroke by this mechanism certainly merit further investigation.

Finally, human clinical studies could be devised to compare chiropractic versus medical or other care in the treatment of various disorders. Such studies could also be employed to compare the efficacy of the various chiropractic techniques. Such studies must involve the use of specific, measurable criteria in both initial and final patient examinations, in order for the data to be believable. In addition, the use of a statistical method appropriate to the type of research design being employed is critical to proper evaluation of the data (25).

Study Designs for Chiropractic Research

Since the first edition of this textbook, a number of chiropractic research efforts have involved the use of "placebo" or "sham" adjustments or other controls for the psychosomatic factor in research (see Chapter 13). As previously mentioned, to demonstrate that correction of the chiropractic subluxation by use of chiropractic adjustment can alter the normal course of the disease, "dis-ease", or disorder in question is essential. Hypothetically, such a sham manipulation would have no substantial affect on the disease (dependent variable) but would appear to be of value to the patient, while chiropractic adjustment (independent variable) would have a substantial curative influence. In this way, the patient would be unable to differentiate between a corrective adjustment and a sham manipulation or treatment (i.e., between the fake treatment and the proposed corrective treatment).

The use of blinds and controls in research is not new, but it is a true challenge to chiropractic researchers faced with an enormous amount of unknowns and variables. Before research can be initiated, the problem being investigated has to be defined, and defining the intervertebral subluxation in a meaningful way has been the enigma of chiropractic clinical research methodology.

According to classical medical research methodology, designs involving multiple, double, or single blinds (26, 27) as well as comparative treatment or a sham (placebo) manipulation (28–30) are advocated. Criteria are established so that each patient included in the study has the same problem (31). Various degrees of impairment or of dysfunction are measured before and after adjustment, by independent observers and by objective reproducible means (31). Patients are not told whether they are receiving corrective or fake manipulations or treatments. Hence, such studies are called double-blind (Figure 14.1).

Center and Leach (20) have offered an alternative to this research approach; this alternative involves the use of the single subject research design. With this design, the patient is his own control for the efficacy of the treatment and is monitored continuously both clinically and physiologically (e.g., galvanic skin response, EMG studies, etc.) before, during, and after intervention with the independent variable (Figure 14.2). Advantages to the use of the multiple baseline design across subjects include its elimination of the need for a sham manipulation and its applicability in small research settings.

Sham Manipulation

A procedure that resulted in the characteristic popping or audible sound of manipulation without effect may be impossible to

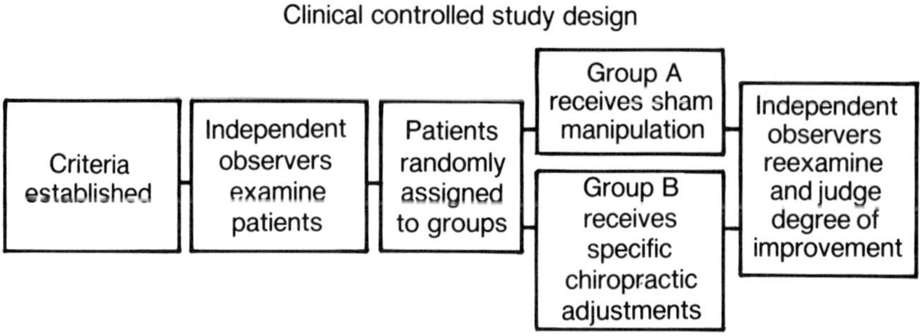

Clinical controlled study design

Figure 14.1. In the clinical controlled study design, as few as two chiropractors and one medical doctor could comprise the independent observer panel. These observers would not know which patients were assigned to control (group A) or adjustment (group B) groups. They would, therefore, be blinded. The patients would not be told whether they would receive specific chiropractic care or simulated care, which would constitute the other blind. One chiropractor would provide adjustments for both groups (giving appropriate adjustment and/or sham adjustment to patients in each group). (Adapted from Buerger AA: Clinical trials of manipulation therapy. In Buerger AA, Tobis JS (eds): *Approaches to the Validation of Manipulation Therapy.* Springfield, IL, Charles C Thomas, 1977, pp 313–319 (29).)

devise (32), but a number of alternatives may be available. For example, mobilizing procedures such as motion palpation can be compared with specific chiropractic adjustment (33). Sham manipulations in chiropractic research have included gentle prodding at the trapezius ridge along the cervicobrachial junction (in studying the effect of thoracolumbar manipulation on arterial flow in the lower extremity) and a nonspecific contact of the adjuster's fingertip with the gluteal area (in researching the effect of "basic technique" adjusting for an antihypertensive response) (34, 35). Finally, chiropractic adjustment may be compared to physiotherapy, analgesics and bed rest, exercise and "back school" (advice concerning proper lifting, etc.), and sham physiotherapy (e.g., detuned diathermy) (Figure 14.3).

Discussion

Certainly, chiropractic research has made great strides in the past two decades. This trend needs to continue if chiropractic research is to lead the profession. The modern patient seeks care that has been tested against all other forms of treatment by utilization of rigorous and objective clinical trials. The federal government expects such research before chiropractic health care

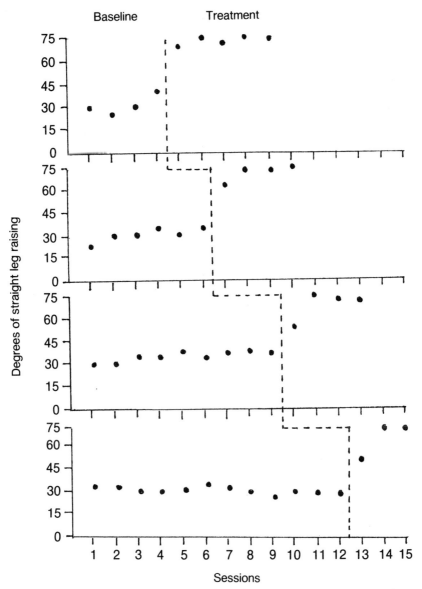

Figure 14.2. An alternative to the use of blinds and sham manipulation is found in the multiple baseline design across subjects which was proposed recently by Center and Leach. In this design, the patient acts as his own control and is monitored objectively before, during, and after intervention. Once a steady state for the dependent variables has been established for the first patient, the intervention treatment is introduced. After the treatment effect on the first patient is established, the intervention treatment is applied to the second patient, etc. This study design has been used extensively by clinical psychologists and educators and, to a lesser extent, by psychiatrists and physical therapists. In this example, the patients are being monitored for improvement in straight leg raising during pretreatment (baseline) and treatment sessions. (Adapted from Center D, Leach RA: The multiple baseline design across subjects: proposed use in research. *J Manip Physiolog Ther* 7:231–236, 1984 (20).)

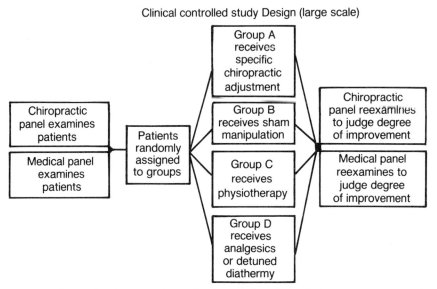

Figure 14.3. This large-scale study design for clinical chiropractic research allows chiropractors and medical doctors to examine and evaluate subjective and objective improvement separately and independently. In this study, some patients could receive either effective or sham manipulation, and others, either effective or sham physiotherapy (detuned diathermy with no current flowing). Obviously, other therapies could be substituted for Groups C and D. (Adapted from Buerger AA: Clinical trials of manipulation therapy. In Buerger AA, Tobis JS (eds): *Approaches to the Validation of Manipulation Therapy.* Springfield, IL, Charles C Thomas, 1977, pp 313–319 (29).)

can be introduced into health maintenance organizations (HMOs) and the military. The media demands that objectivity be the principle of any study. With interdisciplinary and intradisciplinary comparative studies, such demands can be met.

Reliability and reproducibility are critical factors in clinical chiropractic research as well as in medical research. It has been established that reliability diminishes as the volume and the range of data increase (36). Hence, measurement and treatment procedures should be kept simple. Another important concept with regard to chiropractic research methodology concerns selection of patients for the research. Patients should be selected who will classically not respond well to suggestion (as evidenced by the Minnesota Multiphasic Personality Inventory), to ensure that the adjustment itself physically corrected the problem (37, 38). Obviously, such patients are excellent candidates for studies in which

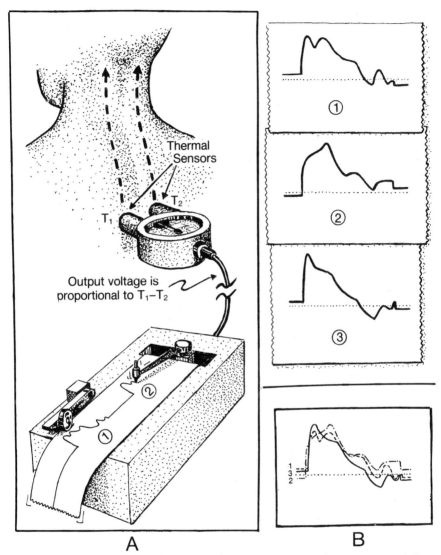

Thermal
Sensors

T_2

T_1

Output voltage is
proportional to T_1-T_2

①

②

③

1
3
2

A   B

Figure 14.4. Illustration of a device for determination of temperature differential along the spine. The hand-held device is moved vertically over the vertebral bodies, and a graph records the difference in temperature from both sides of the spine (A). Each graph (B) represents 6 to 7 seconds of vertical travel; these graphs were recorded at 5-second intervals. The examination was begun at the first dorsal level and ended with a pressure contact at the base of the occiput for a split second. The graphs are shown diagrammatically; the readings were taken by the author after only 1 month of experience with this apparatus. The collage of the graphs shows the reproducibility that even an "amateur" can demonstrate. Use of this technique by chiropractors to determine neuromuscular activity, however, is being replaced somewhat by infrared thermography.

the dependent variable is well defined and easily measured; pain-rating scales are also of help and may be used as predictors of candidates likely to respond to treatment in future studies (39). That a firm diagnosis is not possible in the majority of patients with back pain suggests that all aspects of the condition be researched (40, 41). For example, initial and follow-up disability questionnaires may be used as predictors of outcome (patients tend to respond to treatments in proportion to their scores on certain disability questionnaires).

Evaluation of chiropractic techniques will help determine which are most efficient in correcting the various subluxations and conditions in various individuals. These studies will assist the profession in determining the validity of certain clinical tools as well (e.g., heat reading instrumentation such as is demonstrated in Figure 14.4). Evaluation of chiropractic analysis and diagnosis will aid in all other areas of chiropractic research and treatment. Studies in which chiropractic is compared with medical and other treatments will be more complicated to design, staff, and finance than studies of chiropractic only; these studies are, nevertheless, a top priority in this author's opinion. Conversely, there appear to be no obstacles to the basic chiropractic research which has already begun.

Summary

Chiropractic research is underway on a broad scale at the University of Colorado (2-9). Chiropractic studies have been performed in several areas of clinical investigation, and in these studies, modern research methodology and sham manipulation and controls have been utilized (21, 33-35). The use of the single subject research design (multiple baseline design across subjects) is mentioned briefly, along with its advantages for the small clinic research setting (20). Finally, the use of personality and disability questionnaires, pain-rating scales, and various chiropractic research possibilities are discussed (37-41).

References

1. Suh CH: Lecture presented at the Life Chiropractic College on April 6, 1978.
2. Kelly PT, Luttges MW: Electrophoretic separation of nervous system proteins on exponential gradient polyacrylamide gels. *J Neurochem* 24:1077-1079, 1975.
3. Luttges MW, Kelly PT, Gerren RA: Degenerative changes in mouse sciatic nerves:

electrophoretic and electrophysiological characterizations. *Exp Neurol* 50:706–733, 1976.

4. MacGregor RJ, Oliver RM: A general-purpose electronic model for arbitrary configurations of neurons. *J Theor Biol* 38:527–538, 1973.

5. MacGregor RJ, Sharpless SK, Luttges MW: A pressure vessel model for nerve compression. *J Neurol Sci* 24:299–304, 1975.

6. Sharpless SK: Susceptibility of spinal roots to compression block. In Goldstein M (ed): *The Research Status of Spinal Manipulative Therapy*. Washington, DC, Government Printing Office, 1975, pp 155–161.

7. Suh CH: The fundamentals of computer aided X-ray analysis of the spine. *J Biomech* 7:161–169, 1974.

8. Suh CH: Researching the fundamentals of chiropractic. In Suh CH: *Proceedings of the 5th Annual Biomechanics Conference on the Spine*. Boulder, CO, University of Colorado, 1974, pp 1–52.

9. Triano JJ, Luttges MW: Nerve irritation: a possible model of sciatic neuritis. *Spine* 7:129–136, 1982.

10. Goldstein M (ed): *The Research Status of Spinal Manipulative Therapy*. Washington, DC, Government Printing Office, 1975.

11. Buerger AA, Tobis JS (eds): *Approaches to the Validation of Maniuplation Therapy*. Springfield, IL, Charles C Thomas, 1977.

12. Korr IM (ed): *Neurobiological Mechanisms in Manipulative Therapy*. New York, Plenum, 1978.

13. Haldeman S (ed): *Modern Developments in the Principles and Practice of Chiropractic*. New York, Appleton-Century-Crofts, 1980.

14. Haldeman S: The International Society for the Advancement of Clinical Chiropractic and Spinal Research, 18672 Dodge Ave, Santa Ana, CA 92705.

15. The Foundation for Chiropractic Education and Research (FCER), 1916 Wilson Blvd, Arlington, VA 22201.

16. The Foundation for the Advancement of Chiropractic Tenets and Science (FACTS), 1901 L St NW, Suite 800, Washington, DC 20036.

17. Hildebrandt RW: Scientific journal indexing and its effects on the chiropractic profession. *J Manip Physiolog Ther* 4:1–4, 1981.

18. McDowell FH: Clinical research areas requiring further study. In Goldstein M (ed): *The Research Status of Spinal Manipulative Therapy*. Washington, DC, Government Printing Office, 1975, pp 309–310.

19. Haldeman S: Basic principles in establishing a chiropractic clinical trial. *ACA J Chiropractic* 12:S33–S37, 1978.

20. Center D, Leach RA: Multiple baseline design across subjects. *J Manip Physiolog Ther* 7:231–236, 1984.

21. Vora GS, Bates HA: The effects of spinal manipulation on the immune system. *ACA J Chiropractic* 14:S103–S105, 1980.

22. Haldeman S: The clinical basis for discussion of mechanisms of manipulative therapy. In Korr IM (ed): *The Neurobiologic Mechanisms in Maniuplative Therapy*. New York, Plenum, 1978, pp 53–75.

23. Giles LGF: Vertebral-basilar artery insufficiency. *J Can Chiropractic Assoc* 22:112–117, 1977.

24. Kleynhans AM: Complications of and contraindications to spinal manipulative therapy. In Haldeman S (ed): *Modern Developments in the Principles and Practice of Chiropractic*. New York, Appleton-Century-Crofts, 1980, pp 359–384.

25. Cambell RC: *Statistics for Biologists*. Cambridge, Cambridge University Press, 1974, pp 6–7.

26. Berqquist-Ullman M, Larsson U: Acute low back pain in industry. *Acta Orthop Scand [Suppl]* 170:1–117, 1977.

27. Wymore AB: Chairman's summary: comments on therapeutic studies. In Goldstein M (ed): *The Research Status of Spinal Manipulative Therapy.* Washington, DC, Government Printing Office, 1975, pp 307–308.

28. Kane RL, Fischer FD, Leymaster C: Manipulating the patient: a comparison of the effectiveness of physician and chiropractic care. *Lancet* 1:1333–1336, 1974.

29. Buerger AA: Clinical trials of manipulation therapy. In Buerger AA, Tobis JS (eds): *Approaches to the Validation of Manipulation Therapy.* Springfield, IL, Charles C Thomas, 1977, pp 313–320.

30. Glover JR, Morris JG, Khosla T: Back pain; a randomized clinical trial of rotational manipulation of the trunk. *Br J Ind Med* 31:59–64, 1974.

31. Doran DML, Newell DJ: Manipulation in the treatment of low back pain: a multicenter study. *Br Med J* 2:161–164, 1975.

32. Greenman P: Discussion of clinical observations and emerging questions. In Korr IM (ed): *The Neurobiologic Mechanisms in Manipulative Therapy.* New York, Plenum, 1978, pp 77–89.

33. Wiles MR: Observations on the effects of upper cervical manipulations on the electrogastrogram: a preliminary report. *J Manip Physiolog Ther* 3:226–229, 1980.

34. Wickes D: Effects of thoracolumbar spinal manipulation on arterial flow in the lower extremity. *J Manip Physiology Ther* 3:3–6, 1980.

35. Dulgar G, Hill D, Sirucek A, Davis B: Evidence for a possible anti-hypertensive effect of basic technique apex contact adjusting. *ACA J Chiropractic* 14:S97–S102, 1980.

36. Nelson MA, Allen P, Clamp SE, DeDombal FT: Reliability and reproducibility of clinical findings in low back pain. *Spine* 4:97–101, 1979.

37. Dennis MD, Greene RL, Farr SP, Hartman JT: The Minnesota Multiphasic Personality Inventory. *Clin Orthop* 9:125–130, 1980.

38. Lawlis GF, Mooney V, Selby DK, McCoy CE: A motivational scoring system for outcome prediction with spinal pain rehabilitation patients. *Spine* 7:163–167, 1982.

39. Lehmann TR, Brand RA, Gorman TWO: A low back rating scale. *Spine* 8:308–315, 1983.

40. Roland M, Morris R: A study of the natural history of back pain part 1: development of a reliable and sensitive measure of disability in low back pain. *Spine* 8:141–144, 1983.

41. Roland M, Morris R: A study of the natural history of low back pain part 2: development of guidelines for trials of treatment in primary care. *Spine* 8:145–150, 1983.

Appendix

*I*n the chiropractic literature, it is generally accepted that subluxations are a cause of nerve root compression or irritation and that this lesion ultimately results in various types of dysfunction. A scan of the classic chiropractic literature, however, reveals that, with few exceptions, other etiologies of nerve root compression are generally underemphasized or overlooked (1–5). Moreover, entrapment neuropathies of the peripheral nerve trunks and roots are well documented in the medical literature but, until recently, had been widely ignored in the chiropractic literature (1–29). In many patients, peripheral entrapment neuropathies may generate symptoms that mimick nerve root compression. The chiropractor should be able to differentiate between the two in order to better understand the parameters of his or her effectiveness in managing the patient (differential diagnosis enables the practitioner to determine whether chiropractic treatment should be attempted or whether referral to another provider is needed). A method for noninvasive clinical differentiation between diseases of peripheral nerves and disease of the nerve roots is shown. The method for differentiation between these and diseases of the muscles or spinal cord are also discussed, and the various neuropathies are briefly explored. In addition, the disc lesion and friction fibrosis are discussed, since they are important factors in the etiology of spinal pain.

Differential Diagnosis

Nerve root diseases can be differentiated from other types of disease in several ways. Diseases involving the nerve roots generally produce pain, muscle atrophy, fasciculations, sensory symptoms, flaccid weakness, and other indications that the distribution of signs is segmental (indicating ventral root involvement) or cutaneous (indicating dorsal root involvement) (10, 11, 21, 28).

Spinal cord pathways should be fully functional. Reflexes (deep tendon and superficial) are diminished or absent within the affected dermatome. If the pain and symptoms do not follow the course of the dermatomal innervation, a peripheral nerve lesion should be suspected (10, 11, 21, 28).

Similar to nerve root disease, disease involving the peripheral nerves produces a flaccid-type weakness and atrophy. Sensory findings, however, fall within the same distribution as the motor findings. Thus, there is a combination of motor and sensory symptoms and signs. Also, there may be fasciculations within the distribution of the involved nerve. Although deep tendon and superficial reflexes may be only diminished in nerve root disease, they are absent within the distribution of a peripheral nerve that is affected. When sympathetic fibers are involved, there may be alterations in skin temperature and sweating. Many nerves (poly-neuropathies) or a single nerve (mononeuropathy) may be involved, with the latter being the case with entrapment neuropathies (e.g., compression of the median nerve in the carpal tunnel (carpal tunnel syndrome)).

The most significant characteristic of muscle disease is weakness and atrophy of the involved muscles. There are usually no fasciculations, and there are no indications that the long fiber systems of the spinal cord are damaged. The neural apparatus is intact, so spasticity is absent and reflexes are preserved. Voluntary movement is functional. As the atrophy increases, reflexes diminish (10, 11, 21, 28).

In contrast to the other types of disease just discussed, spinal cord lesions result in damage to the sensory and motor fiber systems of the CNS. Upper-motor-neuron lesions result in spastic paralysis, and lower-motor-neuron lesions result in flaccid paralysis. Increased deep tendon reflexes and a positive Babinski sign are noted in the former. If there is a brain stem or brain lesion, mental status and cranial nerve function may be altered. The level of the offending lesion may be determined by deep tendon reflexes, stretch reflexes, and observation of flaccid weakness and sensation (10, 11, 21, 28).

Neuropathies

There is an almost endless number of ways in which peripheral nerves can be involved in disease processes. As previously mentioned, chiropractors generally focus on osseous entrapment or irritation of the nerve root as a result of subluxation. Yet bacteria, viruses, tumors, fractures, chemicals, and muscles and ligaments may affect the peripheral nerves well beyond the intervertebral foramen (6, 10, 11, 13, 14, 21–23, 27–29). In addition, exostoses or bone spurs as well as a host of other insults may affect the nerve root in the foramen, even in the absence of subluxation there (6, 8, 10–12, 14–21, 23, 27–31). For example, deformities of the dural pouches and strictures of the dural sheaths have been implicated as a cause of nerve compression even when the corresponding apophyseal joint has not been subluxated (19, 30). The following is a list of possible causes of generalized polyneuropathies involving both roots and peripheral trunks:

A. Caused by vitamin or mineral deficiency or metabolism
    1. "Alcoholic neuritis" (vitamin B complex deficiency)*
    2. Beriberi (thiamine deficiency)*
    3. B_{12} deficiency (cyanocobolamin)
    4. Cancer with cachexia
    5. Chronic bacillary dysentery
    6. Chronic colitis
    7. "Chronic progressive polyneuritis"
    8. Diabetes*
    9. Hematoporphyrinuria
    10. Hunger edema
    11. "Korsakoff's psychosis" (polyneurotic psychosis)
    12. Myxedema
    13. Pellagra (niacin deficiency)
    14. Pernicious anemia
    15. Pernicious vomiting
    16. Pregnancy
    17. Pyridoxine deficiency (isoniazid therapy)
    18. "Recurrent polyneuritis"
    19. Senility with cachexia
    20. Sprue
    21. Tuberculosis with cachexia
B. Caused by viruses
    1. Acute rabic myelitis
    2. Chickenpox

---

* Notable common neuropathy.

    3. Encephalomyelitis
    4. Epidemic encephalitis
    5. Erythroedema
    6. Hepatitis
    7. Herpes zoster*
    8. Infectious mononucleosis
    9. Measles
  10. Parotitis
  11. Poliomyelitis
  12. Smallpox

C. Caused by bacteria, bacteriotoxins
    1. Acute enteric fever
    2. Chorea
    3. Diptheria
    4. Erysipelas
    5. Focal infections
    6. Gonorrhea
    7. Influenza
    8. Malaria
    9. Meningitis
  10. Paratyphoid fever
  11. Pneumonia
  12. Puerperal fever
  13. Relapsing fever
  14. Rheumatoid arthritis
  15. Rheumatic fever
  16. Scarlet fever
  17. Septicemia
  18. Serum sickness
  19. Typhoid fever
  20. Typhus fever

D. Caused by chemical toxins
    1. Arsenic
    2. Aniline
    3. Carbon bisulfide
    4. Carbon monoxide
    5. Carbon tetrachloride
    6. Chloral, chlorbutanol
    7. Dinitrobenzene
    8. Ethyl alcohol

9. Ethyl iodide
10. Furadantin therapy
11. Lead
12. Mercury
13. Methyl alcohol
14. Penicillin (accidental injection)
15. Phosphorus
16. Sulfonethylmethane
17. Silver
18. Trichloroethylene
19. Triorthocresyl phosphate
20. Trinitrotoluene

E. Familial
1. Hereditary sensory neuropathy (Denny-Brown Syndrome)
2. Peripheral neuropathy and spinocerebellar degeneration
3. Peroneal muscle atrophy (Charcot-Marie-Tooth-Hoffman syndrome)
4. Progressive hypertrophic interstitial (Déjérine-Scottas syndrome)
5. Refsum's disease
6. Roussy-Lévy syndrome (variant of Friedreich's ataxia)
7. Amyloidosis
8. Tangier disease
9. Porphyria (acute intermittent)

F. Autoimmune
1. Amyloidosis

G. Unknown
1. Lupus erythematosus

H. Neuromuscular junction
1. Myasthenia gravis
2. Botulism
3. Pseudomyasthenic syndrome of Eaton and Lambert

These categories and those that follow are adapted from Turek's, *Orthopedics: Principles and Their Application* (Philadelphia, Lippincott, 1967).

Localized mononeuropathies that the practitioner will want to be familiar with include the following:

A. Caused by mechanical forces
   1. Entrapment neuropathies of the nerve roots
      a. Tumors—malignant, benign neoplasm, lymphoma, etc.
      b. Edema—directly after trauma
      c. Arthritis—spondylitis deformans, osteoarthrosis, etc.
      d. Fibrosis—deformed dural pouches, root sleeve fibrosis
      e. Fracture
      f. Disc protrusion, disc herniation
      g. Spina bifida
         1. Bony lesion
         2. Myelomeningocele
         3. Aberrant mesenchymal structures
      h. Arachnoid cysts, arachnoiditis
      i. Spur formations (osteophytes, exostoses)
      j. Vascular disease which produces nerve root symptoms
      k. Infection of the intervertebral disc which mimicks root compression
      l. Diseases producing kyphosis (resulting in foraminal encroachment)
         1. Disease producing wedged vertebrae (Gaucher's disease, Padget's disease, rickets, malignancy, hyperparathyroidism)
         2. Spondylitis deformans
         3. Compression fracture
         4. Morquio's disease
         5. Hurler's disease
         6. Achondroplasia
         7. Neurofibromatosis
         8. Poliomyelitis
         9. Muscular dystrophy
   2. Entrapment neuropathies of the nerve trunks
      a. Upper extremities
         1. Axillary nerve entrapment
         2. Median nerve entrapment (causalgia, carpal tunnel syndrome)*
         3. Radial nerve entrapment (Saturday night palsy, crutch palsy)
         4. Ulnar nerve entrapment (olecranon groove)* (traumatic ulnar neuritis)

   b. Thoracic outlet syndromes (brachial plexus)
      1. Cervical rib syndrome
      2. Anterior scalene syndrome
      3. Costoclavicular syndrome
      4. Hyperabduction syndrome
      5. Upper brachial plexus (Erb-Duchenne syndrome)
      6. Lower brachial plexus (Déjérine-Klumpe syndrome)
      7. Long thoracic nerve (serratus anticus weakness)
   c. Lower extremities
      1. Sciatic nerve entrapment
         a. Primary nerve disease (inflammatory, degenerative, metabolic)
         b. Secondary nerve involvement (tumors, infection, trauma including pelvic fracture)
         c. Reflex nerve pain (tumours, trauma including back strains)
      2. Obturator nerve irritation (hernia, pelvic dislocation or arthritis, obstetric trauma)
      3. Iliacus compartment compression
      4. Saphenous nerve entrapment (subsartorius fascia)
      5. Lateral femoral cutaneous neuropathy (meralgia paraesthetica)*
      6. Peroneal nerve entrapment (head of fibula)*
      7. Tarsal tunnel syndrome (medial plantar nerve)
      8. Tibial nerve (necrosis of anterior tibial nerve due to pressure buildup in the anterior tibial compartment)
   d. Malposition syndromes
      1. Occipital neuralgia
      2. Abdominal cutaneous nerve entrapment
B. Caused by infectious processes
   1. Diptheria
   2. Tetanus
   3. Streptococci
   4. Leprosy

Of particular interest to the chiropractic theoretician are the entrapment neuropathies of the nerve trunks. These neuropathies may be due to compression of soft tissue structures (e.g., saphenous nerve compressed by the subsartorius fascia) and may be totally unrelated to subluxation (27). More importantly, however, these conditions should be recognized and monitored carefully.

The chiropractor must judge, based on the condition, pathogenesis, chronicity, and state of the patient, whether or not other health care providers should be consulted. In any case, the patient is notified of the possibility of an extra spinal lesion.

Disc Lesion and Friction Fibrosis

From the Medical literature, there can be little doubt that the most often repeated cause of nerve root compression or involvement is herniation or protrusion of the intervertebral disc. In one study at the Mayo Clinic, disc protrusion in the lumbar spine was found to be the cause of 53 of 100 consecutive cases of root pain (14). Lindblom and Rexed (25) documented histologically the effects of 60 nerve root compressions in 160 cadaver specimens. They concluded that the compressions were caused by dorsolateral protrusions of lumbar intervertebral discs. McRae (26) recognized that disc protrusions occur relatively frequently, but he believed that they seldom produce symptoms. Cover and Curwen (12) believed that the "disc lesion" diagnosis is made too often. Hadley (23) is one of the few roentgenologists to state that disc protrusions are not the major cause of compression of the nerve root. His studies—more than any others—have documented the role of subluxations in the production of nerve root compression. Meanwhile, Frykholm (30) found 25 cervical disc protrusions in 20 of his patients. Echols and Rehfeldt (15) failed to identify any ruptured discs in 32 separate operations for sciatica. In general, however, the medical community continues to recognize herniated disc as the most common cuase of nerve root compression. This is a touchy point for some chiropractic theoreticians. They point out that subluxation can place undue stress on the disc, especially when scoliosis is involved (23). Moreover, many chiropractors view the entire pathogenesis of disc prolapse or herniation as an event secondary to subluxation and as a functional breakdown of the articulating facets (4, 5). Although disc protrusions are studied frequently, little thought has been given to the cause of the protrusion. As a result, the medical authors implicate degenerative joint disease (osteoarthritis), including degeneration of the disc, trauma, and aging, as the important factors (11, 23, 28). These are assumptions, however, and have not been proven scientifically. Thus, although the medical community generally regards disc protrusion and the disc lesion as the most common cause of nerve root compression, chiropractors generally believe that disc protrusions are secondary to the pathogenesis of subluxation. Clearly, studies will be needed to resolve this conflict.

Another theory to gain credibility in the medical literature recently is the friction fibrosis theory presented most notably by Frykholm (18, 30, 31) and Sunderland (32–34). Sunderland, a neurologist at the University of Melbourne, recognizes that various changes that narrow or constrict the intervertebral foramen (subluxation, osteophytes, disc herniation, thickening of the ligamentum flavum, etc.) may not actually compress the nerve roots (32).

> The anatomy of the foramen and its contents suggests that reduction in the dimensions of the foramen would need to be considerable before the nerve complex would be compressed. Moreover, nerve tissue tolerates slow compression reasonably well.
>
> The arrangement favors friction fibrosis and the formation of adhesions, induced by the repeated movement of the nerve complex over or against periforaminal pathology of the type outlined above, as a more likely cause of nerve involvement and the development of symptoms.

His studies (see also Chapter 6) documented the susceptibility of nerve roots to stress. In earlier works, Frykholm documented the phenomenon of friction fibrosis in both cadaver studies and operations (31):

> The experiments have shown that if radicular nerve lies in an eccentric position in its foramen and is closely approximated to one of the pedicles[,] it will rub against the bone when the head is moved in different directions. This may be the explanation of the root sleeve fibrosis.

Frykholm hypothesized that this friction caused even more narrowing of the root pouch, which in turn resulted in greater angulation of the nerve roots and more friction between the roots and the dural lining. Thus, the new concept is that the nerves are more susceptible to friction fibrosis and adhesion formation than to compression (see also Chapter 6).

Discussion and Summary

It should be evident that there are many neuropathies with which the chiropractor may be faced. Some of these obviously will be beyond the scope of his or her practice. Others should be monitored carefully while subluxations are being corrected, to note whether the condition is improving or digressing. The purpose of this appendix has not been to downgrade clinically the importance of the subluxation; rather, it has been to upgrade the importance of other neuropathies and disorders unrelated to the subluxation complex and pathology.

References

1. Homewood AE: *The Neurodynamics of the Vertebral Subluxation*. St Petersburg, FL, Valkyrie Press, 1979.
2. Pharoah DO: *Chiropractic Orthopedy*. Davenport, IA, Palmer School of Chiropractic, 1956.
3. Verner JR: *The Science and Logic of Chiropractic*. Brooklyn, Cerasoli, 1941.
4. Gonstead CS: *Seminar of Chiropractic*. Mt Horeb, WI, published privately, 1974.
5. Valentini E: The rate of success of chiropractic management in lumbar herniated discs. *Ann Swiss Chiropractic Assoc* 4:79–86, 1969.
6. Boyd W: *A Textbook of Pathology*. Philadelphia, Lea & Febiger, 1970.
7. Boyes JG: Subluxation of the carpal navicular bone. *South Med J* 69:141–144, 1976.
8. Breig A, Marions O: Biomechanics of the lumbosacral nerve roots. *Acta Radiol [Diagn] (Stockh)* 1:1141–1160, 1963.
9. Brodsky AE: Low back pain syndromes due to spinal stenosis and posterior cauda equina compression. *Bull Hosp Joint Dis* 36:66–79, 1975.
10. Chusid JG: *Correlative Neuroanatomy and Functional Neurology*. Los Altos, CA, Lange, 1973, pp 104–131, 324–333, and 382–393.
11. Curtis, BA, et al: *An Introduction to the Neurosciences*. Philadelphia, Saunders, 1972.
12. Cover AB, Curwen IHM: Low back pain treated by manipulation. *Br Med J* 705–707, March 1955.
13. Derian PS, Bibghaus AJ: Sciatic nerve entrapment by ectopic bone after posterior fracture-dislocation of the hip. *South Med J* 67:209–210, 1974.
14. Eaton L: Pain caused by disease involving the sensory nerve roots (root pain). *JAMA* 177:1435–1439, 1941.
15. Echols DH, Rehfeldt FC: Failure to disclose ruptured intervertebral disks in 32 operations for sciatica. *J Neurosurg* 6:376–382, 1949.
16. Epstein JA, Epstein BS, Lavine LS, Carras R, Rosenthal AD, Sumner P: Lumbar nerve root compression at the intervertebral foramina caused by arthritis of the posterior facets. *J Neurosurg* 39:362–369, 1973.
17. Epstein JA, Epstein BS, Lavine LS, Carras R, Rosenthal AD, Sumner P: Sciatica caused by nerve root entrapment in the lateral recess: the superior facet syndrome. *J Neurosurg* 36:584–589, 1972.
18. Frykholm R: Cervical epidural structures, periradicular and epineural sheaths. *Acta Chir Scand* 102:10–20, 1951
19. Frykholm R: Deformities of dural pouches and strictures of dural sheaths in the cervical region producing nerve root compression. *J Neurosurg* 4:403–413, 1947.
20. Von Reis G: Pain in the distribution-area of the 4th lumbar root. *Acta Psychiatr Neurol [Suppl]* 36:1–135, 1945.
21. Greenfield JG, Blackwood W (eds): *Greenfield's Neuropathology*. London, Edward Arnold, 1976.

22. Grogono BJS: Injuries of the atlas and axis. *J Bone Joint Surg* 36B:397–410, 1974.
23. Hadley LA: *Anatomico-Roentgenographic Studies of the Spine.* Springfield, IL, Charles C Thomas, 1964, pp 230–263 and 422–477.
24. Hadley LA: Intervertebral joint subluxation, bony impingement and foramen encroachment with nerve root changes. *Am J Roentgenol Rad Ther* 65:377–402, 1951.
25. Lindblom K, Rexed B: Spinal nerve injury in dorsolateral protrusions of lumbar discs. *J Neurosurg* 5:413–432, 1948.
26. McRae DL: Asymptomatic intervertebral disc protrusions. *Acta Radiol* 46, 1956.
27. Rob C, May AG: Neurovascular compression syndromes. *Adv Surg* 9:211–234, 1975.
28. Vick NA (ed): *Grinker's Neurology.* Springfield, IL, Charles C Thomas, 1976.
29. Watson-Jones R, Wilson JN: *Fractures and Joint Injuries.* New York, Churchill Livingstone, vol 1, 1976.
30. Frykholm R: Cervical nerve root compression resulting from disc degeneration and root-sleeve fibrosis. *Acta Chir Scand [Suppl]* 160:1–149, 1951.
31. Frykholm R: The mechanism of cervical radicular lesions resulting from disc degeneration and root-sleeve fibrosis. *Acta Chir Scand* 102:93–98, 1952.
32. Sunderland S: The anatomy of the intervertebral foramen and the mechanisms of compression and stretch of nerve roots. In Haldeman S (ed): *Modern Developments in the Principles and Practice of Chiropractic.* New York, Appleton-Century-Crofts, 1980, pp 45–64.
33. Sunderland S, Bradley KC: Stress-strain phenomena in human spinal nerve roots. *Brain* 84:124, 1961.
34. Sunderland S: Mechanisms of cervical nerve root avulsion in injuries of the neck and shoulder. *J Neurosurg* 41:705–713, 1974.

Index

Page numbers in *italics* denote definitions of terms